the
clever
gut
diet

the
clever
gut
diet

Dr. Michael Mosley

ATRIA BOOKS

New York • London • Toronto • Sydney • New Delhi

The information contained in this book is provided for general purposes only. It is not intended as and should not be relied upon as medical advice. The publisher and authors are not responsible for any specific health needs that may require medical supervision. If you have underlying health problems, or have any doubts about the advice contained in this book, you should contact a qualified medical, dietary or other appropriate professional.

ATRIA
BOOKS

An Imprint of Simon & Schuster, Inc.
1230 Avenue of the Americas
New York, NY 10020

Copyright © 2017 Parenting Matters Ltd.
Originally published in Great Britain by Short Books as *The Clever Guts Diet*
Published by arrangement with Short Books Limited

First Atria Books hardcover edition September 2017

ATRIA BOOKS and colophon are trademarks of Simon & Schuster, Inc.

For information about special discounts for bulk purchases, please contact Simon & Schuster Special Sales at 1-866-506-1949 or business@simonandschuster.com.

The Simon & Schuster Speakers Bureau can bring authors to your live event. For more information or to book an event, contact the Simon & Schuster Speakers Bureau at 1-866-248-3049 or visit our website at www.simonspeakers.com.

Manufactured in the United States of America

10 9 8 7 6 5 4 3 2 1

Library of Congress Cataloging-in-Publication Data

Names: Mosley, Michael, author.
Title: The clever gut diet : how to revolutionize your body from the inside out /
   Dr. Michael Mosley.
Other titles: Clever guts diet
Description: New York : Atria Books, [2017] | Revision of: Clever guts diet /
   Dr. Michael Mosley. | Includes bibliographical references and index.
Identifiers: LCCN 2017028069 (print) | LCCN 2017029571 (ebook) |
Subjects: LCSH: Gastrointestinal system—Diseases—Diet therapy—Recipes. |
   Detoxification (Health) | Cooking (Natural foods) | BISAC: HEALTH & FITNESS /
   Healthy Living. | HEALTH & FITNESS / Weight Loss. | HEALTH & FITNESS / Diets.
Classification: LCC RC816 (ebook) | LCC RC816 .M67 2017 (print) | DDC 612.3/2—dc23
LC record available at https://lccn.loc.gov/2017028069

ISBN 978-1-5011-7273-1
ISBN 978-1-5011-7275-5 (ebook)

All disease begins in the gut.

Hippocrates of Kos,
the father of modern medicine

CONTENTS

Introduction

Although this book has "diet" in its title, it is not really about losing weight. That may well happen, if you eat the foods and do the things I recommend, but that's not its primary purpose. *The Clever Gut Diet* is a "diet" in the same way you might talk about being on a vegetarian diet or a Mediterranean diet. It's not about calories or restriction; it's about the sort of food and lifestyle changes you should make if you have gut problems, or simply want to keep yours in good condition.

The gut is not a glamorous organ. When I was at medical school many of my fellow students wanted to study the brain, as neurosurgeons, or become cardiologists, experts in the heart. I never heard anyone say they wanted to dedicate their life to the gut. And yet it is extraordinary—a part of the body, hitherto relatively unexplored, with which I have recently become rather obsessed. Thanks to a huge amount of new research, probing the world within our guts is changing our understanding of the way our bodies work.

As well as extracting energy from our food, the gut accounts for most of our immune system and produces more than two dozen hormones that influence everything from our appetite to our mood.

I also love the fact that, buried in our intestines, deep inside its tissue, is a very thin layer of brain. It's called the enteric system and it is made up of the same cells, neurons, which are found in the brain. There are over one hundred million neurons in the gut, as many as you would find in the brain of a cat. Except, instead of being in one big lump, like the brain on top of your neck, the neurons in your gut are spread out in a thin mesh that extends all the way from your throat to your rectum. This "second brain" doesn't do much geometry or worry about tax returns, but it does orchestrate digestion and moderate gut pain.

When we talk about having "gut feelings" or "gut instincts" we are reflecting the reality of how closely our guts and brains are entwined. In this book I am going to be talking a lot about the "gut-brain axis" and the new science that surrounds it.

Your gut is a wonderful piece of engineering and I hope, after you have read this, you will share my enthusiasm for it. But in many ways the star of the digestive show is not actually part of the human body at all—it is the 2 to 4 pounds of microbes that live in your gut and make up the microbiome.

Until recently the world of the microbiome was a dark, dank, and private one. Down there live creatures that have never seen the light of day, more than fifty trillion of them, at least one thousand different species, a richer diversity of life than you would find in a rain forest.

As is often the case with new scientific discoveries, a lot of genuine research has been misinterpreted and findings have been exaggerated. And, just as these microbes were previously ignored, now they are in danger of being seriously overhyped. Recent research shows that we are not "90 percent bacteria" and "10 percent human," as many books and articles have claimed, but more like 50:50.[1]

In fact, according to one of the researchers who helped explode this myth, the proportions are so similar that "each defecation may flip the ratio to favor human cells over bacteria."

More important, while there are foods that will help your microbiome thrive (and that's why this book contains recipes), few of the products that are sold on this basis have credible science behind them. When it comes to prebiotics, probiotics, and supplements, I will show you what works and what doesn't.

Our widespread ignorance about the microbiome arises from the fact that, until quite recently, its inhabitants, microbes, were impossible to study. We knew they helped protect the gut from dangerous invaders, that they synthesized a few vitamins, and that they gobbled up fiber that our bodies couldn't digest.

Now we know they do far more than that:

1. They help regulate our body weight. As we'll see in later chapters, the microbes in your gut can decide how much energy your body extracts from the food you eat; they control hunger signals, they help decide which foods you crave, and they determine how much your blood sugar spikes in response to a meal.

11

Can your microbiome make you fat? It certainly can. Can you change your microbiome so it works with you rather than against you? You certainly can, and I will show you how.

2. The microbiome not only protects our guts from invaders, it teaches and regulates our entire immune system. Over the last half century we have seen a massive rise in allergic diseases, such as asthma and eczema, caused by an overactive immune system. We have also seen a huge surge in autoimmune diseases, ranging from inflammatory bowel disease to type 1 diabetes, which again are primarily caused by an immune system that has gotten out of control. I will show you how changing the mix of bacteria in your gut can reduce the impact of these diseases.

3. The microbiome takes the bits of food our body can't digest and converts them into a wide range of hormones and chemicals. These, it seems, can control our mood, as well as our appetite and general health. Changing your biome may reduce anxiety and lessen depression.

The tragedy is that, in our ignorance, we have been laying waste to our microbiome and its population of microbes, or "Old Friends." They've been given that name because they have evolved with us over millions of years, and also because so many of them are essential to our health. Just as we have ravaged the rain forests and consigned numerous animal species to oblivion, so we have decimated the populations that live inside us. Fortunately we can help these Old Friends bounce back. I will show you how.

I will also be looking into the latest treatments for a number of gut problems, ranging from gluten intolerance to irritable bowel syndrome. These are diseases that many people struggle with, in part because doctors are often bad at both diagnosing and treating them. They are frequently dismissed as "psychosomatic"—that is, the product of anxiety or depression.

The same used to be said of stomach ulcers. Also known as gastric ulcers, these are open sores that develop on the lining of the stomach and small intestine.

Back in 1994, when I made a television program about ulcers (which I unimaginatively called *Ulcer Wars*), they were common and considered incurable. It was widely believed that they were caused by stress, which made your stomach produce too much acid, and that was what did the damage. The standard medical advice was to eat bland food, change your stressful lifestyle, and take a drug to reduce acid production. If that didn't work, and it often didn't, you might find yourself in the hands of surgeons having parts of your stomach and small bowel removed.

But in Perth, Western Australia, there were a couple of doctors who did not think that stress was the real cause of ulcers. They argued that most ulcers were the result of infection by a previously unknown bacterium that they had identified and named *Helicobacter pylori*.

To make his point, in 1984 one of the scientists, Dr. Barry Marshall, brewed up a flask of *Helicobacter* and swallowed it. A few days later, as he smilingly told me, he started vomiting. He had himself endoscoped; a small tube was passed down his throat and into his stomach. Samples of his now inflamed stomach lining were removed. These showed that his stomach had been colonized by *Helicobacter*.

Barry's wife, Adrienne, who worried that he would become seriously ill, insisted that he stop the experiment. So Barry took a handful of antibiotics, which he had previously shown could kill *Helicobacter*, and soon his stomach was back to normal.

Ten years later, and despite extensive research showing that a short course of antibiotics could cure stomach ulcers, most of the experts I interviewed for my film dismissed Barry's work out of hand. One told me he refused to believe a major breakthrough could have come out of an "academic backwater like Perth." A gut expert who reviewed my film in the *British Medical Journal* described it as "onesided and tendentious."

Normally you make a documentary, it goes out, and that is that. Not with *Ulcer Wars*. I received tens of thousands of letters (these were the days before the internet or email) from people in terrible pain, who had not responded to standard treatments. I ended up sending out thousands of fact sheets, describing the science and Barry's antibiotics protocol.

I still have some of the letters I got back, including one

from a guy called Brian whose ulcer was not responding to standard treatment and who had been told to give up the high-powered job he loved and have most of his stomach removed. He took my fact sheet to his doctor, and begged for a course of antibiotics. His doctor reluctantly agreed and within a couple of weeks he was completely cured. He wrote to me regularly afterward to say he was still going strong.

The tide slowly turned and I was delighted when Barry Marshall and Robin Warren won the Nobel Prize for Medicine for their work in 2005. Looking for and treating *Helicobacter* infection when people have gastric ulcers is now completely standard practice.

The point I'm making is not that antibiotics are the solution to everything. They aren't and their overuse has created other serious gut problems. Nor am I suggesting that stress doesn't matter. It does, and I will show you proven ways to de-stress.

The point is that many diseases have been dismissed as psychosomatic simply because doctors haven't had the right tools to investigate them properly. In the 1930s asthma was treated by psychotherapy because of the mistaken belief that it was "all in the mind." Autism and schizophrenia were once blamed on poor parenting.

One reason I've written this book is that I'm convinced that many common gut conditions are better treated by a change in diet than by drugs or antidepressants.

The initial chapters provide an overview of the gut, which I have written in the form of a journey through my own intestines. These chapters include not only what the gut does, but also what happens when it goes wrong.

Chapter 3 introduces us to the wonderful world of the microbiome and some of the more influential tribes that you will find down there.

Subsequent chapters look at the unexpected ways in which our microbiome influences us, before moving on to scientifically tested ways to keep it in good shape. And finally there is a section of recipes from nutritional therapist Tanya Borowski and general practitioner Clare Bailey.

I've learned a great deal that has surprised me, and gotten a lot of practical benefit from researching this book. I now eat a much wider range of foods, including fermented foods I'd never tried before. I've thoroughly enjoyed the journey. I hope you do, too.

Part I

1

Down the Hatch

As I stood there in the Science Museum in London I began to wonder if this really was such a great idea. In a moment of exuberance I had agreed to take part in a live event at the world-famous museum. I'd said I would swallow a small pill-shaped camera, linked via sensors on my body to a giant screen, so that an audience of hundreds of people would be able to explore, along with me, the intimate, alien world of my gut.

During my medical training and more recently as a television host, I had taken part in some pretty bizarre and painful experiments, but nothing quite like this. In preparation I had fasted for thirty-six hours and taken some powerful laxatives. This was to ensure that the camera would have as clear a view as possible when it got to the murkier parts of my digestive system.

I realized that once I had swallowed the camera I would have no further control of it—how long it would take to work its way through my guts was anybody's guess. We know that food can take up to three days to travel from lips to exit, sometimes even longer. I expected that, because I

17

had drunk four quarts of laxative the night before, my pill cam would travel rather more quickly than normal. But my audience had been warned that if they were waiting for the camera to pop out the other end they could be in for a very long wait.

The camera I had to swallow was smooth and oblong, a bit more than a quarter inch long, the size of a large vitamin pill. Considering the fact that it houses the equivalent of a film crew, complete with lights and camera, it is impressively small. But still a bit of a gulp. It's one of the tools that is normally used by gastroenterologists to go to the parts of their patients that endoscopes and colonoscopes can't reach.

When everything was set up, I swallowed the pill cam, with the help of a glass of water. Down it went, past my tonsils and into my esophagus, beaming live pictures as it traveled. When you swallow food, the esophagus detects it as it touches its wall and the muscles begin to contract, pushing the food farther down. The contraction is so powerful that in theory you could eat while standing on your head.

That was what was supposed to happen. In fact, the camera got stuck at the bend where the esophagus meets the stomach.

I had a moment of panic when I wondered whether I would end up in surgery having my gullet operated on, but fortunately after jumping up and down on the spot for a few moments the camera navigated the narrowing and dropped into my stomach.

Seeing your stomach from the inside, via a fish-eye lens, is an unusual experience. Down there is a cavernous, exotic landscape—pulsing and throbbing with movement. It was pink and pulsatile, a place of slobber and rawhide. When it is empty, the mucosa that lines the stomach is thrown up in folds like a boggy marsh. It reminded me of the surface of Mars. Except slimier. And much more active.

The walls of the stomach are constantly on the move, contracting and folding in on themselves. If the camera had been digestible it would have been pounded and mashed into fragments, then dunked in gastric juices as acidic as a car battery. This acid bath is there to destroy any harmful bacteria or parasites that you swallow along with your food.

In some people, the highly acidic contents of the stomach can leak back up into the esophagus. Known as acid reflux, this can be very painful as it tends to burn the lining. It is commonly treated with acid-suppressing drugs. (If symptoms are mild, ginger tea can help—infuse a couple of slices of fresh ginger in hot water for about thirty minutes. Drink it before a meal.)

Interestingly, it wasn't a camera that gave us the first real insights into our digestive workings. It was, instead, a terrible accident.

The story began in June 1822, when a young Canadian boatman, Alexis St. Martin, working on the shores of Lake Michigan, was accidentally shot in the chest. The blast ripped through his ribs, his lungs, and the front wall of his stomach. Parts of his undigested breakfast started pouring out of his body, along with bits and pieces of his torn stomach. The first person on the scene was a young army doctor named William Beaumont. He dressed the wound, but things didn't bode well and he really didn't expect Alexis to live. Still, survive he did—and in doing so he laid the foundations of our modern understanding of the guts.

Alexis's original wound was huge, about the size of a man's palm, high up on the left side of his chest. We tend to think of the stomach as lying somewhere in the middle, down by the belly button, as that is where a lot of the gurgling noises and stomach pains seem to come from, but it's actually much higher up, right below the diaphragm. The giant hole in his chest shrank, but never fully closed, leaving an opening leading directly from the outside into his stomach. An opening, or hole, like this is known as a fistula.

This was obviously unfortunate for Alexis St. Martin, but a great opportunity for William Beaumont to study the living digestive system in a way that no other surgeon or physician had ever been able to do before.

To keep Alexis close, Beaumont employed him as his handyman and embarked on a series of investigations that went on for nearly ten years.

He would wrap up food in muslin bags—bits of vegetable or meat—and then pop them directly into Alexis's stomach via the fistula. He would leave the bag for a while, then pull it out to see what had happened. A bit like brewing a cup of tea.

As well as putting things into the hole in Alexis's stomach, Beaumont sucked out juices. And it was these experiments that proved to be truly revolutionary, because they turned popular beliefs about digestion on their head.

At that time, the early years of the nineteenth century, it was assumed that digestion was purely mechanical, the muscles in the stomach mashing up the food. Beaumont showed that this was not true. Digestion was also a chemical process. He discovered, for example, that the juice he sucked out from Alexis's stomach was full of hydrochloric acid, which is highly corrosive. He also discovered that these juices were full of digestive enzymes that could break down food if they were mixed together in a bowl.

What happens when you eat and drink

I was keen to see some of this activity going on in my own stomach, so with the camera still in place I ate a meal of steak, French fries, and vegetables, washed down by a glass of apple juice.

I was soon watching, along with my enthralled and slightly disgusted audience, the food and drink that I'd just swallowed arrive in my stomach. The liquid swiftly ran down the walls to the bottom of the stomach, where it joins the small intestine. This is known as the gastroduodenal junction. Down there is a muscular valve, the pyloric sphincter, which acts like a bouncer at a night club, deciding who or what is allowed to pass. When the sphincter is contracted, closed, it holds the food you've eaten in your stomach, allowing the digestive juices and mechanical pounding to do their work. Once it decides that something has been sufficiently pulverized, it opens up and allows it to pass into your duodenum. The whole process has to be carefully orchestrated, which is why you have so many brain cells down there.

Anyway, after a brief pause, the pyloric sphincter decided the apple juice I'd drunk was okay, so it was allowed to pass into my small intestine, like water emptying out of the bath.

There is a useful lesson here for anyone who wants to lose weight: Don't drink your calories.

Unlike those in food, the calories we consume in the form of drink don't fill us up, and some of the worst offenders are the treats which people fondly imagine are healthy. In particular we've been sold the idea that fruit juice and smoothies are good for us because they come from a natural source and contain vitamins. The truth is, unless they are freshly made, they are not a great source of nutrients. What they are good at—the main reason they are so popular—is delivering a very rapid sugar hit to your brain.

You drink the juice, it goes down the hatch, swiftly through your stomach and into your small intestine where the sugar is extracted and absorbed into your bloodstream and transported to your brain. Your brain releases the "feel-good" hormone, dopamine, and you get that familiar sugar kick. Yeah! Give me more of that stuff.

The surplus energy from all that sugar has to go somewhere, and unless you burn it off quickly by doing lots of exercise, it will be stored as fat, either in your liver or around your gut. There are around 120 calories in a small cup or carton of apple or orange juice, the equivalent of five teaspoons of sugar. It may be "natural" but it is still sugar and your body will treat it like Coca-Cola. Store-bought smoothies have similar levels of sugar to fruit juice, some even higher. Drop for drop, grape juice is the worst of the juices, with a single cup containing as much sugar as four doughnuts.

Can you run it off through exercise? Yes, but many people underestimate how much extra exercise they have to do to burn off the calories contained in a small treat.

You may think, "Well, in that case I'll have one of those drinks with zero-calorie sweeteners that I've seen advertised everywhere." Sadly, the evidence is mounting that drinking these can lead to inflammation in the gut and an increased risk of obesity. (For more on this, see page 152).

It is far better to train your taste buds to go for something less sweet. When I'm thirsty I stick to tea, coffee, herbal tea, and water. I love chilled fizzy water with flavorings like lemon, lime juice, or just a slice of cucumber.

Although I am not a fan of fruit juice or smoothies, I do enjoy eating fruit, particularly apples and pears, which are less sweet. One of the big differences between eating an apple and drinking it in the form of apple juice is that an apple has far more nutrients and a lot more fiber so it will hang around inside your stomach for a lot longer and you won't get such a big sugar rush. The undigested bits of the apple will also pass through your small intestine and down into your large intestine, where they will help feed your "good" bacteria. More on that later.

The simple message is that while eating an apple will fill you up, drinking apple juice will leave you hungrier and fatter.

Alcohol

While we are on the subject of drink, what about alcohol? What happens when you knock back a glass of wine or beer? Like any drink it swiftly passes into your stomach. If your stomach is empty then the alcohol will irritate the lining, making the blood vessels swell, increasing both the speed with which the alcohol is absorbed into the blood and the amount of it that goes in.

If you have had something to eat before you drink, particularly something fatty, it will line your stomach, acting as a physical barrier to the booze. So instead of passing straight into the blood vessels that line your stomach, the alcohol will pass out through the pyloric sphincter and into your small intestine.

The small intestine is where most alcohol is absorbed. If it goes into your blood by this route, it takes longer to get into your bloodstream, and so to your brain. If you drink on an empty stomach, your brain typically gets a peak alcohol hit somewhere between thirty and sixty minutes later. If you eat something fatty before you start drinking, that peak will be delayed by up to an hour.

Once alcohol hits your brain, it depresses your inhibitory centers. Contrary to what it may feel like, alcohol is not a stimulant. When I drink too much I normally have a short period of uninhibited fun, followed by a slump and a strong desire to go to sleep. Drinking more than a glass or two of wine doesn't make me good company for long. To slow my drinking, I aim to alternate a glass of water with every glass of wine.

With alcohol in your system, your liver now gets to work, busily breaking it down. First it turns it into a mildly toxic substance called acetaldehyde. This then gets converted into vinegar (acetic acid) and eventually into carbon dioxide and water.

It is the buildup of acetaldehyde (which is more toxic than alcohol) that causes flushing and makes hangovers such a painful experience.

Your liver can break down roughly one unit of alcohol an hour. Drink faster than that and you will get smashed. Keep on drinking heavily and you will eventually destroy your liver.

My wife is not a big drinker, which is just as well. If a woman decides to try to match a man drink for drink, she will normally get drunker, more quickly. That is partly because women tend to be smaller, but also because they have less muscle and more body fat. Some alcohol gets absorbed by your muscles, and thus removed from your system, but fat and alcohol simply don't mix.

Hormones also play a part in metabolizing alcohol, and a woman who goes drinking just before she has her period will find less booze will have the same effect.

Does mixing drinks make you drunker? Broadly, no. How drunk you get is mainly down to how much alcohol you drink, though fizzy drinks are an exception. If you decide to start your evening with a glass of champagne (or sparkling wine), the carbon dioxide in the drink will open the pyloric sphincter valve linking your stomach to your small intestine, allowing the alcohol to pass into your system faster, and getting you drunk more quickly.

Although I have given up fruit juice, I still drink alcohol. That's not only because I like it, but because I believe there are health benefits to be had from moderate drinking. More on that later.

Meanwhile, back to my stomach.

Digestion

When we left it I had just eaten steak, fries, and vegetables, along with a glass of fruit juice. The fruit juice passed through my stomach with hardly a pause, and on to my small intestine where it gave me a sugar hit. My "second brain" or enteric system that controls digestion decided to keep the solid part of my meal in my stomach for further processing.

Thanks to the pill cam, which my stomach had obviously decided was a particularly tough bit of gristle that needed a lot of extra pounding, I could watch the whole fascinating process unfold. The solid bits of food were soon being churned up by the muscles in my stomach, while at the same time being doused in gastric juices, which are released at the sight, smell, or even thought of food. It's this combination of movements and chemistry that turns lumps of food into a creamy mush known as chyme.

Chunks of green vegetables would fly past the camera, along with less obviously recognizable white blobby bits of what I assumed must be meat—soon to be broken down into meat fibers. The vegetable I'd eaten, kale, was extremely fibrous, which was why my stomach was finding it hard to process. The French fries, on the other hand, swiftly started to break apart under the action of acid and enzymes. Reduced to a soggy mass, they were the first of the solid food I'd eaten to be passed on to the next part of the digestive process, my small intestine.

Like the sugary drink that had gone before, foods like pasta, potatoes, rice, and bread are low in fiber and rapidly converted into energy. Once they reach your small intestine they are broken down and absorbed to give you a big blood sugar surge. Foods that are rich in protein, fat, or fiber, on the other hand, take much longer to be processed and absorbed.

Cutting back on readily absorbable carbs, like bread, potatoes, and rice, will probably help you avoid big blood sugar surges, and thus prevent weight gain and type 2 diabetes. However, as we shall see, some people are far more sensitive to these sorts of foods than others.

The green vegetable I had eaten hung around in my stomach for a surprisingly long time, as did the steak. It can take a couple of hours for a steak to be digested and give up its nutrients, which is one reason why we talk about having a "second stomach" when it comes to dessert.

If your body hasn't finished digesting your main meal, your brain may still think, "I'm hungry, I could go for a bit of cheesecake." If you eat slowly, taking time over your meal and perhaps pausing after the main course, you will find the desire for a sugary dessert begins to fade.

There's another good reason to linger over your meal, and that is to give your hunger hormones time to kick in.

Appetite hormones

To accommodate a big meal, your stomach has to expand from the size of your fist to something more like the size of your head. That's a forty-fold increase. It used to be thought that the body regulated weight mainly via the stretch receptors in the stomach. As the stomach expands these stretch receptors send signals to the brain telling it that the stomach is full, and it's time to stop eating. But it turns out that appetite control is nowhere near as simple as that. The gut produces lots of different hunger signals, which play a far more important role in how much we eat than the stretch receptors.

Among the different hormones that regulate appetite, there are some that make you hungry and others that tell your brain when you are full.

The main hormone that makes you hungry is ghrelin. The easiest way to remember is to think "gre for greedy." It is secreted by your stomach when it's empty and travels to a part of the brain called the hypothalamus. There it creates that familiar urge to eat. When you go on a diet your ghrelin levels tend to rise, which makes sticking to it that much harder.

The hormones that tell you when you are full include leptin, which is made by your fat cells. Once released, it tells your brain that you have enough fat on board, no need to eat any more. Unfortunately, when you go on a diet, cut your calories, and begin to lose body fat, those fat cells respond by cutting their output of leptin so you start to feel hungry a lot of the time.

Once upon a time it was hoped that a simple way to cure obesity would be to inject overweight people with leptin. It worked well in mice, but not on humans. The problem is that people who have been overweight for a while have often become severely leptin-resistant. They have lots of leptin running around their system shouting "stop eating, you have plenty of body fat," but their brains are no longer listening.

Something similar happens in type 2 diabetes. If you have a diet high in sugar and simple carbohydrates, like pasta or white rice, your blood sugar levels will be constantly spiking. Your pancreas responds to this by producing the hormone insulin, whose job is to bring those sugar levels down. But, like kids who are constantly shouted at, after a while your cells stop responding to insulin.

Your pancreas pumps out more and more, but it has less and less effect on your blood sugar levels. Instead, the insulin causes your body to go into "fat storage" mode (that's one of insulin's other jobs), diverting extra calories away from your muscles and into your fat cells. As your insulin levels rise, you become hungrier, tired, and, of course, fatter. Eventually you may end up as a type 2 diabetic on medication.

Fortunately, there are other hormones whose job it is to suppress the appetite, including one called PYY, which is produced in a number of places, including the stomach and small intestine.

PYY levels go up after you've eaten, which is helpful because PYY not only suppresses the appetite but also delays gastric emptying, which gives your guts more time to absorb the nutrients you've just eaten.

The good news is that overweight people do not seem to develop a resistance to it in the way they do with leptin. The bad news is that attempts to create a weight-loss drug based on PYY have not been successful, largely because of unacceptable side effects, like nausea.

You can naturally boost your levels of PYY by eating protein, which is why I tend to eat eggs or fish for breakfast (their high protein content keeps me pleasantly full and hunger-free for far longer than if I take in exactly the same number of calories in the form of cereal or toast).

You can also boost your PYY by eating more slowly. It takes time for the food you eat to pass through your stomach, reach your small intestine, and then activate those PYY cells. If you wolf down your meal, you will eat considerably more than if you eat in a more leisurely manner.

If you can, eat at a table and not on the run. Try to put your knife and fork down partway through the meal and give your PYY-producing cells time to spring into action.

As I mentioned earlier, one of the depressing things about going on a diet is that as you shed fat, the levels of your hunger hormone, ghrelin, rise. At the same time, the levels of your appetite-suppressing hormones, like PYY, fall. Your body is trying to hold on to fat, sabotaging your attempts to get rid of it. This is an unfortunate leftover from a time long ago when having a thick layer of fat was like having money in the bank, the key to survival through periods when there wasn't much food around.

The fact that the body seems to be so reluctant to give up its fat has led to some pretty apocalyptic claims about dieting, such as that "95 percent of diets fail," or "It is impossible for most people to shed weight and keep it off."

Commonly quoted though it is, "95 percent" is an invented statistic, along the same lines as "We only use 10 percent of our brains." I've tried to find a credible basis for this claim and it simply isn't there.

Yes, there are plenty of diets that fail, in particular the low-fat diets that have been so heavily promoted over the years. But there are others, like the Mediterranean diet, that have very decent track records.

Long-term studies on diets based around Mediterranean eating (a way of eating I am passionate about, for all sorts of reasons—see my book, *The 8-Week Blood Sugar Diet*) have found that, although there can be a bit of weight regain around the six-month mark, if you keep the weight off for a year, there is a good chance of keeping the weight off for many years.[2]

This is corroborated by a recent study done at the University of Copenhagen, which looked at what happens in the long run to your appetite hormones.[3]

In this study they got twenty healthy but obese people to go on an 800-calorie diet for eight weeks. The volunteers lost, on average, 13 percent of their body weight. They were then put on a one-year program, which included psychological and lifestyle support. Contrary to the myth of inevitable weight regain, they kept it off. They all had blood taken to measure the levels of their appetite hormones, both before they lost weight and after a year.

The scientists found that not only did the levels of the hunger-promoting hormone, ghrelin, return to normal, but that those of the hunger-suppressing hormone PYY were 36 percent higher at the end than at the beginning.

This study shows that if you are able to maintain weight loss for a while (and it may mean up to a year), your body will finally "accept" this new weight as normal.

"At this point," Dr. Torekov of the University of Copenhagen points out, "the body is no longer fighting against you, but with you, which is good news for anyone trying to lose weight."

Gastric surgery

I always encourage people to try to lose weight by changing what they eat, but an alternative approach that is becoming increasingly popular is gastric surgery. Shrinking the stomach will almost certainly lead to weight loss, but it is not for the fainthearted.

I have watched only one such operation in my life, and that was enough.

I met the patient Bob, aged thirty-four, just before he had his operation. Bob was hugely overweight and he rarely felt full, no matter how much he ate.

"I have my breakfast," he said, "of toast and a bowl of cornflakes. Lunchtime is normally a couple of chapatis with some chicken or vegetable curry. After lunch, if I'm still feeling hungry, I have another bowl of cornflakes or Weetabix. In the evening I get some fries, a burger, and later on a sandwich. If I'm still feeling a bit peckish I buy a big bag of potato chips and munch away. I just can't get full. I want to eat everything."

Six years earlier he had had a major health scare.

"I was at home, lying down, and the next minute I had this terrible pain in my jaw and in my arm. I knew immediately that there was something wrong. I went to the hospital and they told me that I'd just had a heart attack. I was only twenty-eight at the time, a young man—and yet I was having a heart attack. I was devastated."

Bob went on a low-fat diet but didn't manage to lose weight. He also developed type 2 diabetes. In the hope of curing his diabetes and regaining his health, he went to see a bariatric surgeon.

There are lots of different types of weight-loss surgery. The simplest is gastric banding, whereby the surgeon puts an inflatable silicone band around the top of the stomach, reducing its ability to expand. In the US this procedure is offered to people with a BMI between 30 and 40, or who have type 2 diabetes or high blood pressure.

The idea is that it cuts the amount of food you can eat at one time, giving your PYY cells time to react and tell you that you are now full. It is relatively noninvasive and it is reversible.

But Bob's surgeon felt he needed something more, so he went for a full gastric bypass, which involves the surgeon not only reducing the size of the stomach but also rerouting some of the small intestine. It is more effective but also more dangerous. Some patients get a blockage, which requires further surgery, while others suffer gastric "dumping," resulting in nausea, rapid heartbeat, fainting, and diarrhea.

A recent review found that those who had a gastric bypass lost more weight and two-thirds were able to reverse their type 2 diabetes, compared to one-third of gastric-band patients.

In the first part of Bob's operation, I watched the surgeon create a small pouch out of his stomach, reducing it from the size of his fist to the size of his little finger. The part of his stomach that produces ghrelin was separated, to try to ensure a permanent fall in his ghrelin levels.

The second part of Bob's operation involved attaching his new, smaller stomach farther down his small intestine, to a section known as the ileum. Cells in the ileum secrete PYY. With his ileum so much nearer his stomach, Bob's PYY cells would "see" food and start to secrete the hormone less than five minutes after it had left his stomach.

Six weeks after his operation Bob had lost more than 40 pounds and his blood sugar levels were back to normal, despite his coming off medication. The main thing he found was that he no longer felt hungry all the time; even small portions would fill him up.

"I had a bite of a burger—I couldn't swallow it. I'm keeping to my diet—I'm happy with that and I can stick with that. Family's happy, I'm happy, can't wait to lose more weight."

Summary

- Digestion is a complex process, organized and coordinated by your second brain, the one that runs the full length of your intestines.

- When you have a meal, fluids are the first thing to pass through your stomach and get absorbed. This is great if you've been drinking water, tea, or coffee (rich in antioxidants), but terrible if what you have been drinking is sugar-laden. Then you'll get big sugar spikes, loads of calories, and hunger sensations soon afterward.

- Like sugary drinks, easily digestible carbs, such as bread, potatoes, and rice, are rapidly broken down and absorbed. Being "easily digestible" sounds good, but unless you need the energy immediately (because you are doing lots of exercise) they will also produce a blood sugar spike, followed by a crash.

- Foods that are rich in protein, fat, or fiber (eggs, meat, vegetables, whole grains) are much more slowly absorbed and will keep you fuller for longer. Eating plenty of fiber, particularly if you get it from vegetables and grains, is very important for feeding the "good" bacteria that live in your large intestine. We will find out much more about these Old Friends, and how to keep them happy, later in the book.

2

Into the Small Bowel . . .
and Beyond

Once you pass beyond the stomach you reach the small intestine or small bowel. To be honest, it's not that small, ranging anywhere between 9 and 30 feet long. It's here that your gut really begins to get to work on your food, which has already been reduced by your stomach to creamy chyme—a pulpy fluid consisting of gastric juices and partly digested food. Every few seconds the surface of your small intestine convulses as a muscular, peristaltic wave passes through. These waves serve to mix the small packages of food that the stomach delivers to the intestines in a very controlled way. It's vital that they are well coordinated, otherwise there would be serious blockage farther down.

As the tight folds on the wall of the small intestine churn the chyme in a frantic corkscrew motion, digestive enzymes from your pancreas and gall bladder begin to flood into the gut. These enzymes break down your food in much the same way that the enzymes in laundry detergent break down dirt, making it easier for your body to absorb the nutrients. The bits of food that your body can't digest are sent down the gut to the ever-hungry microbes that lurk in the large bowel.

There are a few microbes in the small bowel, but there are many more farther down.

The pill cam I'd swallowed missed the opportunity to film a lot of this exciting digestive frenzy because my pyloric sphincter, that picky doorman guarding the entrance to the small bowel, stubbornly refused to let it through until almost everything else had passed. This, I thought, showed a remarkable degree of intelligence (you should never allow television cameras to go just anywhere), but it was frustrating.

Finally, though, I got my first look at the inside of my small bowel. It reminded me of the last time I went snorkeling in a bay full of seaweed. It was murky down there, with bits of partially digested food floating around. Unlike the relatively smooth surface of the stomach, this part of the intestine is covered in lots of villi, millions of little fingery projections that make it look a bit like a fluffy towel. Their purpose is to increase the surface area of the gut, thus maximizing the area available for the absorption of nutrients.

It's often claimed that the villi increase the surface area of your gut to "the size of a tennis court," but is it true? Well, some intrepid Swedes from the University of Gothenburg decided to find out.[4]

They took gut samples from healthy volunteers, examined them under a microscope, counted the villi, worked out their surface area, multiplied this by the length of their small intestine, and came up with a figure of . . . 30 square yards. Their conclusion?

"The total area of the human adult gut mucosa is not in the order of a tennis lawn, rather that of half a badminton court."

Something to think about next time you play badminton.

Common diseases of the small bowel

Celiac disease and gluten sensitivity

The importance of the villi becomes clear if you are unfortunate enough to develop celiac disease. This is an autoimmune disease in which the immune system, which should be defending the body against infection, starts to attack and destroy healthy tissue, in this case the villi of the gut.

The trigger for all this destruction is gluten, or rather gliadin, one of the proteins that gluten is made of.

Gluten is found in grains, such as wheat, barley, and rye, though it is also present in most processed food, including things like soy sauce.

If you've ever made bread you will know that when you mix wheat flour with water it produces a sticky mess. It's the gluten in the flour that produces the stickiness and adds elasticity to the dough, which helps it rise when baked.

Gluten is what makes bread delicious, but in some people it also triggers an immune reaction. When they eat gluten their immune system will not only attack gliadin molecules, but also the lining of their gut. The result is inflammation.

This can lead to pain, diarrhea, bloating, and fatigue. Or, like 50 percent of people with the condition, you may have no gut symptoms at all—you may just go along for many years feeling a bit tired and run-down.

I have a niece with celiac disease. She first started to show symptoms when she was only a few years old. She was tired, frail, off her food, and generally lethargic. My anxious brother and his wife took her to see a pediatrician, who assured them that there was nothing to worry about. My sister-in-law had recently given birth to another girl, and for reasons best known to himself, the doctor decided that their older daughter's symptoms were caused by sibling rivalry. He said that no further investigations were needed. Fortunately, my brother and his wife decided to push for a second opinion, got my niece tested, and discovered that she had celiac disease.

The testing itself is quite straightforward. You have a blood test (looking for antibodies), and if that is positive you may have to have a biopsy done of your small intestine.

There are lots of myths about celiac disease. Here are a few surprising facts:

1. *It is common.*
About 1 percent of the population has celiac disease, and rates have soared in recent years. Unfortunately it is often missed. According to the University

of Chicago's Celiac Disease Center, "At least 3 million people in the US are living with the disease—most of them are undiagnosed." They add that it typically takes four years for someone with symptoms to get a correct diagnosis and this delay "dramatically increases an individual's risk of developing other autoimmune disorders, neurological problems, osteoporosis and even cancer."

In the UK it's estimated that there are at least five hundred thousand people with celiac disease who don't know they have it and who've been seeing their doctors for many years complaining about gut problems. According to Celiac UK, the average time it takes to get diagnosed is thirteen years.

2. *It often starts in middle age.*
Although we think of it as a disease of childhood, the most common age to get diagnosed is between forty and sixty. Undiagnosed celiac disease is a relatively common cause of infertility as well as gut problems.

3. *Even if the tests are negative, you may have a problem.*
There are lots of people who don't have celiac disease but who may have Non-Celiac Gluten Sensitivity (NCGS). Symptoms include cramping, bloating, and diarrhea. Unfortunately, it is hard to diagnose, because there are no reliable tests. You arrive at the diagnosis by excluding everything else.

How common is it? In a recent Italian study researchers tested 392 patients who were complaining of gluten-related problems.[5] They found that 26 out of the 392 (6.6 percent) had undiagnosed celiac disease and two (0.5 percent) had a wheat allergy. The rest were put on a gluten-free diet and followed for two years. Those who were free of symptoms after six months—27 people (6.9 percent)—were considered to have NCGS. So it turned out that 14 percent of this group, who thought they had a gluten problem, either had celiac disease or NCGS.

But what about the rest? When they complained about gluten-related problems were they deluded? I've always been skeptical about claims that gluten affects a lot of people; after all, we have been eating wheat for thousands of years. But then I took part in a revealing experiment organized by the University of Worcester in the UK.

The experiment was done for a TV series. We recruited sixty volunteers, including some who thought they had a problem with gluten, and others who were complete skeptics. We asked them to go on a gluten-free diet for six weeks, and keep a detailed record of gut symptoms, like bloating and nausea. We also did extensive blood tests.

The cunning part of this experiment was that we provided them with gluten-free pasta to eat, which we swapped for ordinary gluten-rich pasta for a couple of the weeks. We didn't tell them exactly what we were doing because we didn't want to influence the outcome.

None of the blood tests, which were looking for things like increased inflammation, showed any change. But, and this for me was a surprise, most of our volunteers reported far more flatulence and bloating during the weeks we were slipping gluten-loaded pasta into their diet, and this stopped as soon as we took it out. Once we had revealed the results, many, including former skeptics, decided to continue on a gluten-free diet.

I'm left confused. On the one hand I am still very skeptical about "food intolerances." I recently sent off samples of hair and blood to a range of companies who claim to be able to detect them and they all came back with a long list of foods (eggs, wheat, milk, broccoli, etc.) that apparently I have a problem with. Yet no two companies provided the same list and in some cases, where I had sent in a couple of samples under different names, they came back with different lists.

So I do think there is a lot of snake oil out there. But I also think people can react to foods in ways that modern science is unable to detect.

I recently met Kathy, a young student who used to love pizza, cookies, and toast. She was regularly ill, with bloating, but assumed that this was part of being a girl growing up.

She also got what she describes as "brain fog" and was frequently in a foul mood, which she assumed was her hormones. Then she developed pain in the joints, which her doctor said were "growing pains."

When these got really bad, and the headaches came on, she Googled her symptoms and then put herself on a gluten-free diet. Within days all her symptoms disappeared. She left it a few weeks, tried eating pasta, and all her symptoms came back, magnified.

She's tested negative for celiac disease and wheat allergy, neither of which she has (this is particularly important if you have a blood relative with celiac disease as it has a strong genetic component), so now she's going on an exclusion diet, aiming to remain gluten-free for a good six months before trying it again.

It won't be easy because so many foods have gluten in them. Foods that you have to avoid on a gluten-free diet include anything with wheat, rye, barley, or spelt. That means bread, pasta, cereals, cake, cookies, etc. You'll also need to lay off the beer and read labels very carefully as many processed foods have gluten in them. Even things like salad dressing can contain barley.

Frankly, eliminating these foodstuffs is likely to help you lose weight and make you feel better anyway. But be aware that a lot of foods labeled gluten-free are stuffed full of sugar and other junk to make them more palatable. You should also be aware that bread and breakfast cereals are often fortified with iron and a range of vitamins, so if you cut them out you may want to take a multivitamin to replace them.

Lactose intolerance

Lactose intolerance is another very common digestive problem that begins in the small bowel. Lactose is a natural sugar found in milk and other dairy products.

When you are young, your small intestine produces a lot of an enzyme called lactase, which breaks lactose down into glucose and galactose (both are types of sugar). These are then absorbed into your bloodstream.

Many people lose the ability to make this enzyme as they grow older, so the lactose passes through the small intestine undigested. In the large intestine the lactose is pounced on by bacteria, which will turn it into fatty acids and gases such as carbon dioxide, hydrogen, and the smelly one, methane. It's these that produce common symptoms of lactose intolerance, such as flatulence and bloating.

The easiest way to find out if you are lactose intolerant is through an exclusion diet, along the lines of the gluten-exclusion diet I mentioned above (see more on this in Part II). There are also other, more exotic and expensive ways to find out, which include a hydrogen breath test and a stool acidity test.

Irritable bowel syndrome (IBS)

Irritable bowel syndrome is another incredibly common gut disease, affecting around one in five people at some point in their lives. Symptoms include stomach cramps, bloating, and either diarrhea or constipation. After rumbling on for a while, it often gets worse when people hit their thirties.

Dave is thirty-two years old. He has been constipated for many years, regularly becomes bloated, and has recently begun putting on weight at an alarming rate. He has also begun to experience reflux, where acid from his stomach leaks up into his gullet.

Dave was on what he calls a "beige" diet. He had cereal or toast for breakfast; sandwiches for lunch; pasta, pizza, or fish-and-chips in the evening. Many of his evening meals were quick, rushed, carb-heavy, and eaten late at night in front of the TV.

He went to his GP, who offered him medication, which made no difference. So he went to see nutritionist Tanya Borowski. Tanya has a lot of experience working with people who have IBS, which is why I asked her to provide recipes for this book.

Tanya recommended some simple lifestyle changes, such as cutting down on the booze, taking time for lunch, and not having his meals late at night. She also asked him to commit to being in bed by 10:30 p.m. at least four nights a week. Finally, she offered him a two-stage program which works for most of those with IBS (see page 186).

She suggested that for four weeks he remove wheat from his diet, switch to grains that are browner and less easily digestible, reduce the carbs that cause bloating, and cut out all dairy. At the same time she recommended he increase the amount of color in his diet (see page 120) and have a tablespoon of apple cider vinegar with water before each meal. She thought Dave would also benefit from having some bitter greens to get his digestive juices flowing. To improve his constipation she gave him magnesium citrate and triphala, a traditional Ayurvedic herbal treatment.

After four weeks of more or less sticking to this approach, Dave had lost 9 pounds and was feeling a lot better. The acid reflux had gone, as had the bloating. So it was time to reintroduce some of the foods he had cut out. He started eating cheese again, but this time the proper stuff (see page 138), and he also started on full-fat yogurt and fermented foods (see page 140). She gave him a probiotic to take, too (see page 147).

After another four weeks, Dave was symptom-free and "ready to rock."

The sort of approach I've just outlined is likely to work for most people who have mild IBS, but if it doesn't or yours is more severe, you might need to try something more extreme. The current best-tested approach to treating IBS was developed at Monash University, Australia, and is known as the FODMAP diet. If you are interested, do visit their website for more information (www.med.monash.edu /cecs/gastro/fodmap/).

FODMAP stands for Fermentable Oligo-, Di-, Mono-saccharides and Polyols. These are carbs that cause digestive problems for some people. The FODMAP approach is to cut them all out, then steadily reintroduce them. It is a complicated diet which is best done with the help of a dietician who is FODMAP trained. Visit our website, clever guts.com, for more information on finding a FODMAP practitioner.

The Appendix

Moving on down the gut, we come to the appendix, a worm-like structure that sits just below the junction of the small intestine and the large bowel. Most people are familiar with the appendix, mainly because they know someone who's had it removed due to an infection (appendicitis).

For a long time people thought the appendix was a waste of space, something left over from our distant ancestors. Now we know that it is actually a reservoir for "good" bacteria, ready to be released after a bad bout of, say, food poisoning.

Imagine you have eaten something dodgy and your gut has become infected by some nasty microbes. Your body will unleash a powerful immune response and also try to flush out the bad guys by flooding your gut with fluid. You will experience this as dramatic diarrhea.

Once you've purged your guts you will want, as soon as possible, to reseed them with the "good" bacteria to prevent more bad guys coming in and taking over. That's where the appendix can help. It acts as the Noah's Ark of the gut world, ready to repopulate your gut when the waters subside.

Summary

- Diseases of the small bowel are common and often hard to diagnose.

- Celiac disease affects 1 percent of the population and is often not picked up until middle age. Studies suggest it is now four times more common than it was fifty years ago.

- Gluten intolerance is also on the rise. There is no reliable test and the only way to find out if you have it is by going on an exclusion diet.

- Irritable bowel syndrome affects one in five people. It is best treated by a change in diet.

3

The Kingdom of the Microbiome

Eight long hours after I swallowed it at the Science Museum, my pill camera had traveled just five yards. Although many in my audience had drifted away, others came along to replace them. They were rewarded, around six o'clock in the evening, by the sight of the camera finally escaping from my small intestine and reaching the wide open spaces of my large intestine or colon, home to the legendary microbiome.

Here, for the first time, we could see signs of the alien species that shape our lives in so many unexpected ways. I had obviously seen my biome's relatives many times before; after all, 60 percent of feces is made up of bacteria from the colon and who doesn't, occasionally, examine their stool? But I had never previously encountered them in their natural setting.

The microbes that live in the colon are mainly bacteria, but there are also some fungi, viruses, and simple, primitive animals called protozoa. Together they form a wonderfully complicated ecosystem. These were the creatures that I most wanted to meet.

There are trillions of them down there, so the camera couldn't, of course, pick them out individually, though it did begin to encounter small murky fragments of what is known in the trade as "formed matter," i.e., feces.

Think of the microbiome as a small but incredibly complex rain forest. It throbs with life, hundreds of different competing and coexisting species. We used to think their job was pretty basic: to protect our gut from invaders; to synthesize a few vitamins like vitamin K, which the body doesn't produce itself; and to produce nasty smells while gobbling up the fiber that our bodies can't digest. Now we know they do far more than that.

As I mentioned in the introduction, we know of three other vitally important things that the microbiome does:

1. It regulates your body weight. As we'll see in a moment, the microbes can decide how much energy your body extracts from the food you eat, and much more. Can your biome make you fat? It certainly can.

2. The biome not only protects your guts from invaders but it also regulates your entire immune system. Changing the mix of bacteria in your gut can reduce the number of coughs and colds you get as well as the impact of a range of allergenic and autoimmune diseases.

3. The biome takes the bits of food our body can't digest and converts them into hormones and other chemicals. The study of how the creatures in our guts affect our brains has its own name, "psychobiotics," and is one of the most exciting areas of current biome research.

In the next chapter I am going to cover some of the things you can do to ensure that you and your biome stay healthy. I'm also going to justify some of the claims I've just made, because on the face of it they are quite outrageous. But first, let's meet some of the Old Friends that live in your gut.

The Old Friends

Microbes don't have teeth or claws, let alone arms or legs. But they are brilliant chemists. They can take simple compounds, such as carbon or sulfur, and turn them into an extraordinary number of different chemicals. They use these skills to extract food from unlikely places (bacteria can live on rock and radioactive waste), to destroy competitors (early antibiotics, like penicillin, were created by fungi), and to manipulate us. When it comes to chemistry, the microbes that live in your gut are among the most ingenious of them all.

Although there are hundreds, possibly thousands, of different species living, breeding, and dying in your gut, until recently it was impossible to identify most of them. That's because they won't grow outside the warm, airless environment of your intestines. It would be like bringing fish onto dry land and hoping they'd thrive. So, although we were all flushing billions of bacteria down the toilet, there wasn't much that scientists could do with that valuable material.

Then came the genetic revolution and soon we were able to find traces of bacteria by looking for fragments of their DNA. It's rather like DNA finger-printing, which allows the police to trace criminals even when they are no longer present at the scene of the crime. Instead of relying on eye-witnesses, they can now collect a drop of blood from the crime scene, and with this they are able to create a genetic profile of the offender.

Scientists know which bacteria should be in your gut, and can match what they find in your stool to giant databases of likely suspects. In fact, there are now several companies, including British Gut, American Gut, and uBiome, which will sequence your microbiome for under $100 and provide you with a report of the results.

The process is simple. You go to their website, log on, and send them money. They send you a plastic tube, a spatula, and instructions on how to collect a fecal sample. You put your feces in the tube, give it a good old shake, stick it in the mail, and wait awhile to get the results. If you are not living in the US, expect the whole thing to take at least two months.

I recently sent my feces off to uBiome and the results, when they came back, were certainly interesting. The first bit of information comes under the title, "Body Weight," which gives you an idea of what most people who use the service are interested in.

So what did they find in my gut, and how do the contents compare with the average microbiome?

Firmicutes

One-third of my gut bacteria was *Firmicutes*, which is lower than average. Outside the body, *Firmicutes* do a whole range of things, from fermenting beer and wine to cleaning up toxic waste. Inside your guts one of their main tasks is to help digest the fat in your diet. Once upon a time, when food was less plentiful, this was an incredibly useful thing because it meant people with lots of *Firmicutes* could extract the maximum energy from all the fatty things they ate.

These days having a lot of *Firmicutes* is not such a good thing, and has been linked to a higher risk of obesity. People with high levels of *Firmicutes* tend to be those who live on a typical Western diet (i.e., high in fat and sugar).

Bacteroidetes

Just over half (55 percent) of my gut bacteria was *Bacteroidetes*. This is a good thing, according to uBiome, because having a microbiome tilted in favor of *Bacteroidetes* is associated with a lean body type and with less inflammation in the gut.

This group of bacteria also plays an important role in teaching your immune system how to behave (they help control how violent your immune response is) and in breaking down the undigested fiber from vegetables that makes its way into your colon. When they do this they produce a number of valuable substances, including butyrate.

Butyrate

From our point of view, butyrate is a wonderful chemical. It helps control the growth of our gut wall cells, and that protects us against bowel cancer. It also has powerful anti-inflammatory effects.

Inflammation is one of the ways your body defends itself. If you get the flu you will probably become hot and inflamed, with achy joints, as your body tries to destroy the viruses. That's fine. The problem comes when inflammation persists. Just as having a chronically infected tooth is a bad thing, having persistently inflamed guts can lead to pain, bloating, gas, constipation, and eventually bowel cancer.

One way to counter this is to boost your butyrate levels by eating food with lots of fiber in it. The undigested bits of fiber will reach your colon and give your "good" bacteria plenty to chew on. Well fed, these "good" bacteria will provide you with lots of lovely butyrate.

As well as lowering inflammation, butyrate helps to maintain your gut lining, the barrier that keeps bacteria and other toxins from escaping into your blood. If this barrier starts to break down, you get a condition known as "leaky gut syndrome" which can lead to all sorts of distressing problems, including IBS. (See page 60 for more information.)

The recipes at the back of this book contain foods proven to boost your butyrate levels.

Akkermansia

As well as lots of *Bacteroidetes* I was pleased to see that I had decent levels of a species called *Akkermansia*. *Akkermansia* are unusual because, unlike most of the microbes in your gut, they don't live on the remains of your food. Instead, they live on mucus, the snotty stuff that your gut wall secretes to protect itself against invading bacteria. Like *Bacteroidetes*, *Akkermansia* strengthen the gut wall and reduce inflammation. The more *Akkermansia* you have, the better.

We know this, in part because of a series of recent experiments done by scientists from Belgium, where *Akkermansia* was first identified.[6]

They showed that if they gave *Akkermansia* to overweight mice it stopped them becoming obese and developing diabetes. It even worked when the bacteria had been pasteurized—heated to above 160°F. Willem de Vos, one of the researchers, said, "This came as a complete surprise. Even more surprising was the fact that the bacterium was in some ways more active after pasteurization: not only reducing obesity and diabetes, but preventing these diseases from developing in the first place."

A protein, with the unsexy name Amuc 1100, found on the outer surface of the bacteria, seems to be responsible. Human studies are underway and a company has been created to scale up production of both *Akkermansia* bacteria and Amuc 1100.

In the meantime, you can boost your own levels of *Akkermansia* by eating more polyphenol-rich foods (see the box on page 120), and also by fasting. Since *Akkermansia*, unlike most of the bacteria they have to compete with, are not dependent on the food you put in your mouth (they live, as I mentioned before, on the mucus in your gut wall), they will thrive when you cut down your calories. I recommend intermittent fasting as part of any regimen to boost your gut health. Think of *Akkermansia* as your Fasting Friends. More on this in Chapter 6.

Christensenella

Sadly, what the uBiome people didn't find in my gut was a lovely little bacterium called *Christensenella*. People who have lots of them tend to be lean, despite sometimes rather poor diets.

Zoe Budd is tall and slim. Her feces were recently examined and found to have thirteen times the normal levels of *Christensenella*.

"I have a pretty terrible diet," she told me. "I love croissants, bacon sandwiches, cookies, and cakes." She does try to eat plenty of vegetables but always goes for the pudding and the chocolate cake when given half a chance.

Christensenella seems to be one of those bacteria you inherit from your mother and which only thrive in people with the right genes. It's not clear, if you don't already have them, how you would go about acquiring them. There is no evidence, for example, that consuming them in capsule form will do you any good (although you can buy them on the internet).

Zoe's kids are like her, tall and slim, so maybe they've inherited a few *Christensenella* bacteria, along with half her genes.

Lactobacillus

I was also surprisingly low in *Lactobacillus*. This bacterium lines your intestines and is good at protecting your guts from bad guys, such as the fungal pathogen *Candida albicans*. Many women will be familiar with this nasty little beast because it is responsible for vaginal thrush. *Lactobacillus* destroys pathogens like *Candida* by spraying or injecting them with hydrogen peroxide, the stuff that people use to bleach their hair.

If your *Lactobacillus* are weakened by a course of antibiotics that you have taken to treat something else, this can give *Candida* a chance to take over in your gut. Once it does it is hard to dislodge.

Some strains of *Lactobacillus* are important for mental health; at least those who take it in the form of a probiotic (a capsule containing live bacteria) report that it improves anxiety and mood.

In combination with other probiotics it may also help people with IBS. More on that later.

Bifidobacterium

Finally, one bacterium that I have lots of, in fact three times more than average, is *Bifidobacterium*. These guys break down otherwise indigestible fiber and, like *Lactobacillus*, protect your gut from other less friendly microbes.

You get them early in life from your mother's breast milk, and you will also find lots of them in cheese and yogurt, two of my favorite foods, which could explain why I have so many in my gut. Like *Lactobacillus*, they are a popular probiotic.

Leaky gut syndrome

As well as protecting your gut from attack by unfriendly bacteria, "good" bacteria help reinforce your gut wall, making sure that bad stuff doesn't get out of your gut and into the rest of your body. When that happens you get "leaky gut syndrome."

If you tell a doctor you have leaky gut syndrome he or she will probably roll their eyes and sigh. Many doctors think it is an imaginary condition dreamed up by loopy promoters of alternative medicine to flog dubious supplements to desperate customers. It's certainly what I used to believe.

Yet there is now clear evidence that leaky gut, or "intestinal hyperpermeability," is a real condition. It is characterized by bloating, pain, gas, cramps, tiredness, and food sensitivities, as well as generalized aches and pains.

It occurs following a gut infection, a course of antibiotics, a poor diet, or even a strenuous bout of exercise, when the tight junctions between the cells that form your gut lining start to loosen. Think of the lining as the Great Wall of China, designed to keep invaders out, but which now has some bits missing, through which the enemy can squeeze. Once bacteria and other toxins get out of your gut and into your blood you are in trouble.

Diagnosing leaky gut

A leaky gut can be hard to diagnose, which is why many doctors are so skeptical about its existence. One way is to use a "sugar probe"; this involves giving you a mix of two different types of sugar to drink. One of these sugars must be small and simple, chemically speaking (mannitol), while the other should be bigger and more complex (often lactulose).

In a normal gut the small sugar molecules will be able to squeeze between the gaps in the gut wall, but the large ones won't. If you have a leaky gut even the large molecules will get through, and a much higher ratio of lactulose to mannitol will be detected in your urine.

Recent studies, using sugar probes, have shown that common gut disorders, like IBS, which are often dismissed as being "all in the mind," frequently do have a physical cause.

Understandably, people who have spent years with pain and bloating become anxious and depressed. But antidepressants may not sort them out. A change in diet, to one that particularly encourages the growth of "good" bacteria, just might. See the recipe section at the back of the book for some excellent, soothing broths and smoothies to help repair the gut lining.

The bad guys

As well as microbes that keep your gut healthy, there are plenty of "bad" guys on the prowl, microbes that can cause serious gut problems, given half a chance. I've done a lot of traveling, particularly in some of the poorer parts of the world, so I am personally familiar with quite a few of these.

Campylobacter

This is the most common cause of food poisoning in affluent countries. Symptoms include abdominal pain, severe diarrhea, sometimes with blood, and vomiting. It can lead to IBS and arthritis. It can also cause pregnant women to miscarry.

You typically pick up *Campylobacter* by handling raw chicken or undercooking it. It takes a single drop of juice from a raw chicken to infect someone, and the bacterium is present in the majority of chickens sold in supermarkets.

Washing a chicken before you put it in the oven is a terrible idea because it just spreads the bacteria around. Instead, just make sure you cook it properly.

While most people have heard of *E. coli*, *Salmonella*, and *Listeria*, *Campylobacter* causes more cases of severe food poisoning than those three put together.

E. coli

Many types of E. coli are harmless, but some can cause bloody diarrhea leading to anemia (severe blood loss) and even kidney failure. They are also a common cause of urinary tract infections. You commonly get a gut E. coli infection from eating infected meat that has not been fully cooked (i.e., to at least 160°F). You can also pick it up from drinking raw milk.

Salmonella

Another little delight is Salmonella, the food-poisoning version that causes diarrhea, stomach cramps, and vomiting. Typically symptoms begin within twelve to seventy-two hours of swallowing it and last up to a week. If you become seriously ill you may need to go to the hospital because you could die from dehydration. Salmonella typhi, which causes typhoid fever, is much nastier and more likely to be fatal. It infects over 20 million people, worldwide, every year.

Clostridium difficile (also known as C. diff)

This is one of those bacteria that may well be hanging around in your guts right now, doing little harm, being kept in its place by your "good" bacteria. Then you get a minor infection and your doctor prescribes you a broad-spectrum antibiotic. This wipes out much of your normal gut biome, but leaves *C. diff* intact, because these are tough and normally very antibiotic-resistant bacteria. With their rivals destroyed, *C. diff* may seize the opportunity to take over. It is a bit like the invasion of Iraq: Once the allies had destroyed Saddam, they created the circumstances in which ISIS could thrive.

Once *C. diff* are in charge they are incredibly hard to get rid of. Symptoms include watery diarrhea, fever, and abdominal pain, which can go on for many years. Incredibly, *C. diff* kills some 29,000 people every year in the US and costs around $1.5 billion a year to treat.

Standard treatments, which include yet more antibiotics, are often ineffectual. If this is the case, your best bet may be something that sounds rather unpleasant: a fecal microbial transplant or FMT.

Fecal Microbial Transplant (FMT)

As the name implies, FMT involves doctors taking feces from a healthy donor and squirting it into an infected patient. The hope is that the microbes from the healthy donor will overwhelm and destroy the *C. diff* bacteria. The transplant can be done via a nasogastric tube, but there is a higher success rate if it is done via a colonoscopy and then squirting in the donor stool. The main

downside, apart from being distasteful, is that the donor stool has to be properly screened to ensure it's not harboring anything nasty. I have seen one FMT done and the whole thing took less than thirty minutes. The results were spectacular.

Rose had spent many years in pain, having to rush to the bathroom at all hours of the day and night. There had been countless failed attempts to treat her with antibiotics. Yet she was cured within hours of being given a fecal transplant and was able to return to normal life shortly afterward.

Although it's relatively new, FMT is amazingly successful. Randomized controlled trials have shown that a staggering 94 percent of patients make a full recovery after a single fecal transplant.

The treatment is now being tried out on all sorts of other gut conditions, from IBS to leaky gut syndrome and type 2 diabetes. People have even started doing DIY versions, but this is one procedure I really wouldn't try at home.

In search of diversity

It's not just the type of bacteria in your gut that matters, it's also the diversity. You want your biome to be as multicultural as possible. The loss of a minor species won't have too much impact, but if a few "bad" species, like *C. diff*, begin to take over, the effect can be disastrous. A diverse micro-biome will allow your gut to recover much more quickly from a bout of diarrhea.

Unfortunately, like animals in the wild, many species in our gut are in decline and have been for decades. It's partly because we eat such a narrow range of foods, which means our gut bacteria also have to live on a restricted diet. Of the 250,000 known edible plant species, we use less than 200. Seventy-five percent of the world's food comes from just twelve plants and five animal species. It's one reason why I am going to encourage you to branch out a bit and try things like fermented foods, which you may never have considered before.

Another reason for the decline is the widespread use of antibiotics, not only to treat us but also to help the animals we eat put on weight. Routine use of antibiotics in ani-mals as a growth promoter is now banned in Europe but is still common practice in other parts of the world, includ-ing the US.

Finally, there are emulsifiers. These are chemicals that are added to processed foods to extend their shelf life. They've been shown to reduce microbial richness, and may directly contribute to colitis and diabetes.

How to make your biome more diverse

There is a measure, called the Simpson index, which tells you just how diverse your biome really is. My most recent score was 7.99, which puts me into the top 30 percent of "most diverse microbiomes" among those who have sent stool samples to uBiome. This, however, is not much to brag about. People like the Hadza (a tribe of hunter-gatherers who live in Tanzania) have a biome which is at least twice as diverse as mine.

A couple of years ago Jeff Leach decided to try and acquire a healthier gut and blog about it under the title "Going Feral: my one-year journey to acquire the healthiest gut microbiome in the world (you heard me!)."

His attempts to acquire a healthier gut included hanging upside down under a tree in Africa while someone poured liquidized feces from a Hadza tribesman into his bum via a funnel.

Jeff is not particularly wild or deranged. In fact, he is a very well-respected scientist and cofounder of American Gut. Based at the Knight Lab at the University of California, San Diego, American Gut describe themselves as "one of the largest crowd-sourced, citizen science projects in the country." Like uBiome, for a modest donation, they will take a look at your stool and let you know what is in it.

Things they have discovered so far include:

- The more different types of plants you eat, the more diverse your microbiome.

- People who have at least one alcoholic drink a week have a more diverse microbiome than those who don't drink at all.

In his search for "the healthiest microbiome in the world," Jeff was not about to confine himself to eating a few more plants and having the occasional drink. He decided to move in with the Hadza, adopt their diet, "eating the plants, animals and drinking the same water (with the occasional baboon turd floating in it)," and see what happened.

So what did happen? Well, the initial impact on his gut was a decrease in microbe diversity, although it soon bounced back.

He also saw a big increase in our friend *Akkermansia*. As I've mentioned before, *Akker* is good because high levels of it are associated with low levels of obesity. It also protects you from invasion by nasty microbes by reinforcing your bowel wall. In the weeks he was with the Hadza his *Akkermansia* went from almost nonexistent to being a dominant player.

He thinks there are a number of reasons for this, including the fact that he, like the Hadza, went for quite long periods without food. As he writes in his blog:

"I'm gonna go out on a limb here and suggest that the Hadza—and presumably our ancestors—were periodically fasting . . . I don't mean going all day without food—there's plenty of food in Hadza land. Plenty. But rather they don't immediately solve hunger pangs by opening a bag of chips as it takes just a little bit of effort to get some food and sometimes you delay your desire to eat because of it. This little bit of extra time between mouthfuls is what I mean by intermittent fasting in the case of the Hadza and what I experienced when I was following the diet."

On his blog, humanfoodproject.com, Jeff makes a number of suggestions about what you can do to ensure a healthier biome, in addition to cutting down on the snacks. These include:

1. Avoid antibiotics if you can, because a course of broad-spectrum antibiotics can "take weeks, months or even years for your gut microbial community to bounce back from—if at all."

2. Open a window. We spend 90 percent of our lives living indoors. Studies show that opening a window increases the diversity of microbes in your house and therefore, presumably, in you.

3. Eat more plants. That doesn't necessarily mean giving up meat, nor does it mean simply eating a lot more carrots. It means eating as wide a range of different plants as possible. But it also means eating lots of different bits of the plant, not just the tasty bits. "Consume the entire asparagus, not just the tip. Consume the trunk of the broccoli, not just the crown."

4. Get your hands dirty. Preferably by gardening. This connects you with the trillions of bacteria that live in the soil and is a good way of getting in some exercise.

The end of the pill cam's journey

At the beginning of this chapter, we met Pill Cam, the camera that I swallowed in the Science Museum, just as it entered the kingdom of the microbiome. I got a brief glimpse of that gloomy realm, but the farther the camera went, the murkier the images became. Anyway, by then it was late and the museum was keen to close. So, with little prospect of any more usable footage being beamed back from this strange and alien world, we decided it was time to end the show. The audience went home, and so did I.

Unobserved, the pill cam continued on its merry way, along my large intestine, all 1.5 yards of it, through my muscular sigmoid colon, and into my rectum. Finally, many hours later (about twelve hours, if I remember correctly), it exited my body. You'll be pleased to hear I've cleaned the camera up, polished it, and kept it as a memento of a most unusual day.

In all, it took the pill cam around twenty hours to travel from my lips to the toilet bowl. This is pretty fast going, as a typical transit time (the time it takes from eating to excretion) is, according to the Mayo Clinic, normally more like forty hours. In one study they did with healthy volunteers, they found the transit time in men averaged thirty-three hours, while women took a more leisurely forty-seven hours.[7]

If you are a keen self-experimenter and want to time yourself you could try eating food with red food dye in it and see how long it takes for the dye to appear in your feces.

Summary

- A healthy biome is home to a rich diversity of microbes. It is a delicately balanced ecosystem where bacteria vie for supremacy.

- Some, such as *Lactobacillus* and *Bifidobacterium*, produce substances like butyrate that damp down inflammation. They also protect your gut from attack by unfriendly microbes and help reinforce the walls of your gut, preventing leaky gut syndrome.

- Although too much junk food and overuse of antibiotics may have damaged your biome, you can shift it in a healthier direction by changing what you eat and drink, and by embracing the great outdoors.

- These days you can get your biome sequenced for about $100. This will tell you what's down there and what shape it's in. If you repeat the tests after following some of the advice in this book you should soon be able to tell if the Clever Gut Diet has made a difference, although you will also be able to tell from the scales and how you feel.

4

How Your Biome Influences You, and How You Can Influence It

As we have discovered, a healthy microbiome should be made up of as rich and varied a range of microbes as possible. There are trillions of them down there, and together they add up to roughly the same number of cells as the rest of your body combined (microbes are generally much smaller than human cells).

As I will show you in a moment, they affect things like your mood, your weight, and how active your immune system is. While they influence you, you can also change them. What you eat and the way you live will have a huge impact on the sort of creatures that thrive in your internal rain forest.

But how do you acquire these microbes in the first place?

Where your microbiome comes from

Most of us get our biome from our mothers. When you were in her womb your gut was largely free of microbes. What happened next depends on the way you were born.

If you were born vaginally, you would have traveled down the birth canal and taken a good gulp of your mother's feces and vaginal fluids. With no competition from existing microbes, these bacteria would then have rapidly colonized your guts. Later, if you were breastfed, you would also have acquired "good" bacteria from her breast milk.

If you were born by a Cesarean section (C-section), things would have been very different. The first bacteria you encountered would have been those hanging around in the operating room, those on the skin of the people who held you, and anything else you inhaled or swallowed in the first few hours of life.

Stool samples taken from babies who were delivered by Cesarean section show that they have a very different gut bacterial population from those who were born vaginally.

Does this matter? Yes, very much so. Thanks to a large study done by researchers from the Harvard T. H. Chan School of Public Health,[8] we know that babies who are born by Cesarean section are far more likely to become obese children and overweight adults.

In this particular study, aptly known as GUTS (Growing Up Today Study), researchers tracked more than 22,000 babies from birth into adulthood. They weighed the children when they were teenagers, and again when they were in their twenties.

The results were dramatic, particularly when they compared brothers and sisters. Children born via C-section were 64 percent more likely to be obese than their siblings born vaginally, despite sharing the same genes, being brought up in the same household, and eating the same food. This strongly suggests that it is the gut bacteria that are making the difference.

"Cesarean deliveries are without a doubt a necessary and lifesaving procedure in many cases," said Jorge Chavarro, senior author of the study. "But Cesareans also have some known risks to the mother and the newborn. Our findings show that risk of obesity is another factor to consider."

Cesarean-born babies are also far more likely to develop allergies later in life.

With Cesarean rates currently running at around 26 percent in the UK, 35 percent in the US, 50 percent in China, and up to 80 percent in Brazil, this is storing up problems for the future.

One way around this problem, if a C-section has to be done, is to try and expose the baby to some of its mother's microbes as quickly as possible. It's known as "vaginal seeding" or microbirthing, and involves taking a swab from the mother's vagina and anus, and wiping it over the baby's mouth, eyes, and face shortly after birth.

This approach has its fans, but Dr. Aubrey Cunnington from the Department of Medicine at Imperial College London isn't one of them. He thinks that unless it is done in a carefully controlled way, the potential risks, such as picking up an infection from mom, outweigh any likely advantages.

"One colleague had to intervene when a mother with

genital herpes, who had undergone a Cesarean section, was about to undertake this process," he says. "Swabbing could have transferred the herpes virus to the baby."

He also thinks there are better ways to ensure your baby gets the best start in life. "Encouraging breastfeeding and avoiding unnecessary antibiotics may be more important to a baby's gut bacteria than worrying about transferring vaginal fluid on a swab."

Breastfeeding is certainly going to give a baby's biome a good start and may well contribute to the fact that breast-fed babies are half as likely to develop eczema or asthma as a baby who is exclusively bottle fed.

As well as a good mix of fats, proteins, and carbohydrates, breast milk contains complex sugars which, oddly enough, babies can't digest. It seems that their main purpose is to feed the "good" bacteria which are, hopefully, growing in the baby's gut. The fact that breast milk evolved to feed these Old Friends shows just how important they are.

As we get older our biome changes and the number of species colonizing our gut increases, up from about one hundred species in an infant to around one thousand in an adult. By the time we are three years old, our biome will be largely settled, though it can still change in response to infection, antibiotic treatment, and changes in diet.

Although you can't do anything about the way you were born or how your mother fed you, you can do something about how you currently feed yourself. And your microbiome. Before we come to that, I'd like to dive into some of the many surprising ways in which your microbiome affects you as an adult.

Summary

- Your microbiome is formed in the first couple of years of life and heavily influenced by how you were born.

- Breast milk contains a healthy mix of proteins, fats, and sugars. It also contains compounds that a baby can't digest, but which encourage the growth of "good" bacteria. Oddly enough, breast milk contains substances whose only purpose is to feed Old Friends.

How your biome makes you fat

As we've just seen, being born by C-section has a lasting effect on your gut bacteria and your waistline.

Being exposed to repeated courses of antibiotics when you are a child also increases the risk that you'll become overweight, particularly if those antibiotics are given in the first six months of life.

As an adult there are various ways your particular mix of bacteria may help you put on weight:

1. Some gut bacteria extract more energy from the food you eat than others.

2. They can influence how much your blood sugar levels rise when you eat.

3. They may affect your mood and the food choices you make.

Extracting energy from food

Our digestive systems are not 100 percent efficient. Some of the calories we take in will also get excreted. And, although much of the energy in the food we eat is extracted by our gut, we also depend on our gut bacteria to do some digesting for us. Mice with sterile, bacteria-free guts are much skinnier than normal mice, despite consuming exactly the same calories.

We also know that some bacteria, like *Firmicutes*, are better at extracting energy from the food we eat than others. Which means that if I have more *Firmicutes* in my gut than my wife (which I do), I will probably be excreting fewer calories, after eating exactly the same meal, than she does.

Evidence for this comes from a study done by researchers from the National Food Institute, who collected feces from thirty-two children, half of whom were overweight and half of whom weren't, and gave the samples to mice.

The mice who got feces from the overweight kids gained significantly more weight than those who got it from the slim kids, despite eating the same food. The researchers also measured the unspent energy in the mouse feces and found that those who had put on the least weight were excreting the most calories.[9]

Why weight loss is not simply a matter of eating less and exercising more

What studies like this have done is undermine the idea that has dominated weight control thinking for the last half century: "CICO" (calories in, calories out). According to CICO the reason we're fat is because we eat more calories than we burn off. The answer to obesity is eat less and exercise more.

Except, of course, it's not as simple as that. As we have just seen, the bacteria in your gut can influence how many of the calories that go in, stay in. We have also seen that the gut does not treat all foods exactly the same. Eating cake will not have the same effect on your body as eating steak.

Unlike the steak, the sugar and flour in the cake will be swiftly absorbed, making your blood sugar levels soar. In response to this your pancreas will pump out insulin to bring them down. It will also switch your body into fat storage mode. The energy from the cake will now be stored as fat.

But the surge in insulin is normally followed by a crash in blood sugar levels, which will leave you tired and hungry. Studies show that when this happens you eat more. So you put on weight. That's why it's important to avoid frequent blood sugar spikes.

To do that you need to cut back not just on sugary drinks and snacks, but also on any foods that make your blood sugars surge.

Which ones are these? Well, there is a measure, known as the Glycemic Index (GI), which ranks foods according to their impact on blood sugar levels.

Easily digestible carbs like white bread, rice, potatoes, and pasta have a high GI score, while foods with fiber in them, like broccoli or whole grains, score low. To see a list go to glycaemicindex.com.

Although it is a helpful, and sometimes surprising, guide to what causes blood sugar spikes (who would have thought that a boiled potato would have the same impact as eating a tablespoon of sugar?), the GI is also limited. To create a GI figure for any particular food, ten to twenty volunteers are fed that food and researchers then measure what happens to their blood sugar levels. On the basis of this, they calculate and publish an average GI score.

The problem is that people respond differently to exactly the same foods. The reason? The different mix of bacteria in their guts.

We know this because of a massive study by the Weizmann Institute in Israel, the largest of its kind ever undertaken.

Personalized nutrition

The Personalized Nutrition Study done at the Weizmann Institute is one of the most fascinating studies I have come across, promising, as it does, to create the first truly personalized diets.

For this study, immunologist Dr. Eran Elinav and computer scientist Dr. Eran Segal recruited eight hundred volunteers and ran extensive tests on them. At the start of the study they took blood and stool samples and lots of physical measurements, like height and weight.

The volunteers were also fitted with skin-mounted monitors, which measure blood sugar levels almost continuously. They wore these for a week, while keeping detailed records of everything they ate and drank, as well as how much sleep they were getting and how much exercise they were doing. The Erans wanted to measure, with great precision, the impact their normal daily diet and lifestyle was having on their blood sugar levels.

All in all the scientists collected over 1.5 million blood sugar measurements.

They found, to everyone's surprise, that eating exactly the same foods had very different and often unexpected impacts on people's blood sugar levels. Some volunteers' blood sugar levels soared in response to rice, while for others it had very little impact.

Is chocolate bad for your blood sugar levels? Yes for some, but not for others.

The team used data from the stool samples they'd collected, along with details such as age and gender, to create an algorithm, a computer model that could predict which foods would cause an individual's blood sugar levels to spike.

They then tested their algorithm on a fresh batch of volunteers, comparing their predictions with how people actually responded. So how did it do? Extremely well.[10]

Finally, they recruited yet another group of volunteers, took stool samples, and using this data created a personalized diet sheet containing "good" and "bad" foods for each one of them.

The volunteers were asked to follow their personal diet sheet for two weeks. For one week they had to eat foods the algorithm had predicted would have a bad effect on their blood sugar levels. For the other week they ate only the "good" foods on their list.

It wasn't just salad and vegetables on the "good" list and cake on the "bad." Some people were free to eat chocolate and drink alcohol, while others had to shun apparently healthy food.

According to Eran Segal it resulted in impressive differences. "When they were on the 'bad' diets their blood glucose levels rose, well into the abnormal range, but when they were on the 'good' diet they stayed within the healthy range."

Curious, a friend of mine, Dr. Saleyha Ahsan, went to Israel to try it out.

Saleyha's journey

Saleyha is a busy doctor who is constantly on the go and often doesn't have the time to eat well. She used to be in the army and was incredibly fit, but since damaging her knee she has had to restrict the amount of exercise she does. As a result she has put on a lot of weight, which she was keen to do something about. As she told me, "I've always watched what I eat, but right now I just can't seem to lose the weight. I need help."

For Saleyha it is not just about wanting to look a bit slimmer. She has a family history of type 2 diabetes and knows she is at significant risk of going down that road. She also has polycystic ovary syndrome, which would be helped by losing some fat around her waist.

So she went and spent time with the Erans at the Weizmann Institute. Like all the other volunteers, she was fitted with a glucometer under her skin, so her blood sugar levels could be constantly measured. Her sleep and activity levels were monitored by a wristband, and she was given an app to record her mood and everything that she ate. They also collected stool samples from her, which showed she had high levels of the sort of bacteria linked to obesity and diabetes.

Then she embarked on six days of eating food, provided by the institute, that would test her blood sugar responses.

Finally she was presented with two lists of foods. A green "good" list, which included things like avocados, bananas, and dark chocolate; and a red "bad list," which unfortunately included some of her favorite foods, such as sushi and grapes, which she'd always seen as healthy.

She agreed to eat only the green-listed foods for a month. After three weeks she started to notice a difference. She no longer felt tired during the day and her hunger pangs had gone. Her skin looked better and she had lost 7 pounds.

"I used to blame myself," she says, "for being lazy but now I realize it's not as simple as that. Once I started eating foods that produce less blood sugar spikes I stopped having ups and downs or hunger pangs."

By changing her diet she had also changed the mix of bacteria in her gut. At the end of the month there was a marked fall in the bacteria associated with obesity and diabetes.

It is impractical for most of us to hang around in Israel with glucose monitors trying out lots of different foods to see what happens. So the Erans have created a company to commercialize their work, which is just being launched.

You register, pay, and they send you a kit which you use to collect a stool sample. You also have to fill in a short questionnaire and do an A1C test (this is a blood test that gives an accurate measure of what your blood sugar levels have been for the last ninety days or so—your doctor can do it).

You send these off, they analyze them, and then use their algorithm to produce a personalized nutrition app that recommends specific foods/meals you should eat if you want to keep your blood sugars down. If you stick to the green foods and shun the red ones they are confident that, like

Saleyha, you will lose weight and feel more in control. They see this as the first step toward a truly personalized diet. Early days, but really interesting. To find out more, visit our website cleverguts.com.

To evaluate how effective this approach is, the two Erans have just started another trial in which they will follow a large group of people for a year. The people they've recruited for the trial have prediabetes, which means they are well on the way to developing type 2 diabetes, so it will be an important test of their ideas.

They are certainly not short of volunteers. Previous participants were so enthusiastic about their experience that they have urged friends and family to join in.

Yo-yo dieting

The two Erans are also researching the effect of gut bacteria on yo-yo dieting. As anyone who has ever dieted knows, the big challenge is not so much losing weight as keeping it off. Many people take up a diet, shed loads of fat, plateau, despair, and pile the weight back on.

As we've seen, what makes it particularly hard to keep weight off is that, when you shed fat, your body fights back, using your appetite hormones against you. As your fat cells shrink your body produces more of the hormones that make you hungry and fewer of the ones that suppress appetite. That's the bad news. The good news is that if you tough it out those appetite hormones will reset.

Intriguingly, your microbiome also seems to contribute to the problem of yo-yo dieting.

To find out what's really going on, a team led by the two Erans took mice and fed them till they were really fat. Then the mice were put on a low-calorie diet till they'd reverted to their previous slim selves. The scientists did this several times. At the end the mice looked the same as when they had started.

But they weren't. Given the chance to eat freely, the mice piled on weight, laying down fat faster than they had the first time they had been fed a high-calorie diet. What had happened was that their biome had changed. The new mix of microbes included many that now encouraged weight gain.

"It seems that the microbiome retains a 'memory' of previous obesity," says Eran Elinav. "This new microbiome accelerated the regaining of weight when the mice were put back on a high-calorie diet."

Fortunately, they found a way to reverse this. And that was by feeding the mice flavonoids.

Flavonoids are made by plants to protect themselves against parasites and harsh weather. You'll find them in blueberries, cherries, blackberries, plums, grapes, tomatoes, and green tea. They are powerful antioxidants—and they also encourage your body to burn fat. More on them in Chapter 5.

The Erans showed that yo-yo dieting, at least in mice, creates an unhealthy biome, rich in bacteria that are hell-bent on destroying flavonoids, which in turn leads to rapid weight gain.

When they gave the mice some flavonoids in their drinking water, they discovered that the mice had "reset." They no longer showed accelerated weight gain when put on a high-calorie diet.

The flavonoids the Erans used were apigenin, which is found in parsley, celeriac, and chamomile tea, and naringenin, present in grapefruit, oranges, and tomato skin. It is unlikely that eating those foods will give you as big a dose as the mice got, and it's not even clear if the flavonoids that work for mice will work for us. But they are good foods to eat, so what have you got to lose?

Summary

- Your biome helps determine how much energy you extract from food and, to some extent, how much weight you put on.

- Your biome also influences how much your blood sugar levels respond to particular foods.

- By analyzing stool samples it's possible to predict which foods will make your blood sugars surge. This offers the possibility of a truly personalized diet, based on valid science.

- Eating flavonoids or foods rich in flavonoids may help you avoid regaining weight after a diet.

- More disturbingly, there is evidence that your biome can influence the food choices you make.

The biome and your brain

We like to think that we are in charge of the decisions that we make, from what we decide to eat to where we go on vacation. But the truth is we make a lot of decisions subconsciously, guided by signals and cues that we are not even aware of.

Why did you eat that muffin on the way to work? Was it because you really, really wanted it, weighed up the benefits and the costs, and decided to buy it? Or did you see it when you went into the coffee shop and just pick it up on a whim? Most of us eat mindlessly most of the time, guided by habit and influenced by advertising.

But what about our gut bacteria? Is it plausible that the tiny single-celled creatures lurking in our gut can also influence our decision-making?

I think so, and so do an increasing number of scientists who work in this area. Our microbes certainly have the opportunity, the motive, and the tools to manipulate us.

I've talked before about the second brain in your gut, the enteric system that contains the same number of neurons as you'll find in the brain of a cat (I love that fact!) and which communicates with the brain in your head via the vagus nerve. The vagus nerve is like a busy telephone line, with lots of messages going in both directions. The enteric system talks to your brain and your brain talks back.

There is plenty of evidence that your microbes can hack into this system and talk directly to your brain via the vagus nerve. They also produce a range of hormones and neurotransmitters that reach your brain via your bloodstream.

Dopamine, for example, is well known as a "feel-good hormone." The microbes in your gut produce lots of it, possibly to reward you for doing what they want you to do (like eat more cake). The microbes in your gut also produce chemicals that control your mood, like serotonin and GABA (a neurotransmitter that acts in a similar way to the antianxiety drug, Valium). They even make a range of chemicals that are strikingly similar to leptin, ghrelin, and PYY, the main hunger hormones.

So microbes have means. They also have the motive. Life in your gut is not for the fainthearted. It is a state of endless war. Life down there is nasty, brutish, and short. The microbes are not only competing for space and scarce resources; they also have different dietary demands. Some thrive on sugar, others love fat. The more sugar you feed the sugar eaters, the more they want. They are not like a friendly dog, hanging around waiting gratefully for whatever comes their way. They are fighting for life. They will do anything to give themselves the edge.

"Microbes have the capacity to manipulate behavior and mood through altering the neural signals in the vagus nerve, changing taste receptors, producing toxins to make us feel bad and releasing chemical rewards to make us feel good," says Dr. Athena Aktipis, from the Arizona State University Department of Psychology. She has recently collaborated on a major review of the scientific literature, which asked the question: "Is eating behavior manipulated by the gastrointestinal microbiota?" The answer was a resounding "yes." They put together a convincing case that microbes not only influence how much we eat but what we eat.[11]

They point to research that shows that having a wide range of different species in your gut normally means you are slimmer and healthier. Having a more limited ecosystem is associated with being overweight and sickly.

Why should this be? Well, the argument goes that in a diverse microbiome all those tiny creatures will clamor to be heard, and, like a gang of children shouting at once, they can be ignored. The problem comes when one group—say, the ones who thrive on junk food—start to dominate. As a gang, these bad guys will now be much more influential and, by producing chemical signals, generate cravings for junk food, cravings that you will find hard to resist.

So how sure are we that this actually goes on? At the moment the most convincing evidence that microbes can alter behavior comes from animal studies. It has been known for a long time that mice, when infected by bacteria called *Toxoplasma gondii*, become strangely reckless. Normally a mouse will keep to the shadows and avoid anything to do with cats. But when they are infected by *Toxoplasma* there is a complete change of behavior. They are now attracted by cat urine and will deliberately move out into the open, to be killed. The *Toxoplasma* bacteria are manipulating the mouse's behavior. They want it to be eaten by a cat, so that they can then infect the cat.

Similarly, if you feed feces from mice who display anxiety-like behavior (no one talks about "anxious mice" because we don't know what they are thinking) to mice that don't have *Toxoplasma* in their gut, then those mice start to behave in a more anxious manner.

Scientists have found they can make mice swim for longer, and more doggedly, if they feed them bacteria called *L. rhamnosus*.[12] Furthermore, rather brutally, they found that if you sever the vagus nerve in these mice, so that the gut can no longer talk to the brain, the mice do not change their behavior after being fed these bacteria.

When it comes to humans, the evidence is more circumstantial. In one study involving twenty-two people,[13] half of them chocaholics and the other half indifferent to chocolate, the researchers found that those who loved chocolate had a very different set of microbes from those who weren't interested in anything sweet, despite the fact that both groups had been put on an identical diet.

There was also an impressive double-blind, randomized, placebo-controlled trial in which researchers showed that they could significantly improve depressed people's moods by giving them a probiotic containing a mix of *Lactobacillus acidophilus*, *Lactobacillus casei*, and *Bifidobacterium bifidum*.[14]

Turning their attention to infants, the ever curious scientists found, when they looked into babies' diapers, that children with colic (inconsolable crying) had reduced gut diversity and fewer *Bacteroidetes* (the "good" guys) than children who didn't cry as much. One theory is that lots of screaming means parents are more likely to pay attention, fuss and feed, thereby providing the microbes, which are irritating the baby's guts and causing it to scream, with more food.

A rather spooky suggestion that emerges from all this is that cravings could be catching, jumping from one person to another.[15] Perhaps cravings, and the resulting tendency to put on weight, are not just socially contagious but literally infectious, like a cold.

To be honest I find this a bit far-fetched. I have lived with my wife for more than thirty years and she has shown no signs of being infected by my sweet tooth.

Along with the rather frightening possibilities that this research throws up, there are some consoling thoughts. If cravings really are being generated by a group of cunning bacteria in your gut, then you have it in your power to starve them out.

All you have to do (and I don't underestimate how tough this can be) is keep away from the thing you crave and hopefully the cravings will reduce as those microbes die off. There will be more on this subject in the next chapter.

Summary

- The microbes in your gut can communicate directly with your brain via the vagus nerve.

- They also produce hunger hormones and neurotransmitters which they may use to influence your cravings and your behavior.

- If so, then changing the microbes in your gut may also change your cravings.

Allergies and gut bacteria

Two hundred years ago, life expectancy in the developed world was less than half what it is today. People died young of infectious diseases like typhoid, cholera, and tuberculosis. What they didn't commonly have were autoimmune diseases, like type 1 diabetes, or allergies, like asthma. None of the characters in Jane Austen's nineteenth-century novels ever complains about hay fever or having a food intolerance. Charles Dickens never suggested that Oliver Twist or any of his artful dodger friends suffered from eczema. Allergic diseases are a modern plague, a product of the twenty-first-century lifestyle.

What autoimmune diseases and allergies have in common is that they are triggered by an overactive immune system. One popular theory as to why this occurs is known as the Hygiene Hypothesis. Crudely, the problem is that we are too clean.

The argument goes that because antibiotics and wet wipes have made our environment increasingly sterile, our immune system has responded by becoming overly sensitive. So, rather than just fighting genuine threats, like cholera, it treats things like pollen or gluten, which aren't threats, as if they were. We've cleaned up our world to such an extent that our immune systems, with nothing better to do, have gone on the rampage.

According to the Hygiene Hypothesis, your immune system is a bit like a grumpy teenager, bored out of his skull, who decides to start smashing up the house. The solution? Give him something to do, enemies to fight.

Some people have taken this to mean we should be deliberately exposing our kids to infectious diseases when they are young, while others use this theory to attack vaccinations, arguing that they overwhelm the immune system.

The trouble with the Hygiene Hypothesis is that it is probably wrong and doesn't fit the facts. In recent years it has been replaced by a subtler and more plausible version which focuses on the problem of the Old Friends we met earlier.

According to the Old Friends Hypothesis, the real problem is not that our immune system is bored, but that it is ignorant. Like us, our immune system comes into the world with an awful lot to learn. One of the things it needs to learn quickly is what is dangerous and needs to be fought, and what is okay and should be left alone. You really don't want your immune system launching an all-out attack on the microbes in your gut, since many of them are essential for your health.

In the past the immune system would have been taught these essential lessons by Old Friends, the gut microbes that evolved with us over millions of years.

Sadly, as we have seen, because of the overuse of antibiotics and a diet heavily based on highly processed foods, many of those Old Friends are no longer with us or only present in small numbers.

So the real problem is not that we are exposed to fewer infectious diseases (which are dangerous and harmful) but that we have lost contact with the microbes that evolved with us and without which our immune system just won't function properly. We have lost or accidentally killed off huge numbers of important Old Friends, and that is what is creating the modern problems of allergy and auto-immunity.

The next chapter of this book is all about how you can cultivate and reestablish contact with some of these Old Friends. But before that, I would like to introduce you to a gut parasite that has also evolved with us over millions of years and that has, in the past, played an important role in controlling and educating our immune system. It's not really an Old Friend but it can, in the right circumstances, be a valuable ally. I'm talking about parasitic worms.

Horrible hookworm

The hookworm is an unpleasant bloodsucking parasite that lives in the small intestine. It infects half a billion people worldwide and is a major health hazard in the tropics and subtropics.

Its life cycle is both fascinating and repulsive. It lives in human guts where it meets and mates with other hookworms. The female then lays around thirty thousand eggs a day, which exit the gut in the feces. Protected and fed by all the warm feces, the eggs hatch into larvae and wait patiently for a new host to come along.

If you happen to be strolling by, barefooted, and step on ground that has been infected by the larvae, they will swiftly burrow in through your skin and travel up to your lungs. This will make you do a lot of coughing, which brings them up through your trachea and into your esophagus. You swallow them, they somehow survive the warm acid bath of your stomach and make it to your small intestine. Here they latch on and begin to drink your blood.

Knowing all this, you might wonder why anyone would want to deliberately infect themselves with hookworm. The answer is, if you are desperate enough you will probably try anything.

I met Daniel Hayman in an Indian restaurant, where we both ordered a hot curry. This was something Daniel could never have contemplated doing a few years ago because he has Crohn's, a form of inflammatory bowel disease (IBD). IBD affects about 1.3 million people in the US and, as with most autoimmune diseases, rates are rising. It happens when your immune system, possibly triggered by an infection, starts to attack the lining of your gut wall.

Unlike celiac disease, IBD cannot be treated by the simple removal of an irritant. Like a hooligan who has decided to target your house, it keeps coming back. You may have periods of remission, but it is normally a lifelong condition.

Symptoms of IBD include pain, recurring or bloody diarrhea, extreme tiredness, and weight loss. The first treatment you will be offered is usually steroids to calm things down. If that doesn't help, you may be given medication to suppress your immune system or to reduce inflammation. Some people end up having the inflamed bits of their bowel removed.

Daniel tried to control his disease with conventional medicine, but he continued to feel terrible, so he turned to something very unconventional—hookworm.

Daniel went on the internet and ordered live hookworm larvae from someone who had been cultivating them in his own body. When the larvae arrived Daniel placed them on his skin, where they burrowed in, eventually finding their way to his guts. The improvements were not immediate. In fact, it took almost a year before he felt fully well.

"Were you spooked by the idea of having a parasite inside you?" I asked him.

"Not at all," was his surprisingly calm reply. "I believe that human beings have evolved to have plenty of parasites inside them. It's part of life. You should try it."

And then, just to prove how far he had come, he dug into one of the hottest curries on the menu. He is, he assured me, no longer afraid of food. "I'm finally free. Thanks to the worms I can eat pretty much anything I want."

So what's going on? I met up with Helena Helmby, from the London School of Hygiene and Tropical Medicine, who studies how worms interact with the immune system.

"We have a sophisticated immune system," she told me, "that's constantly on watch. But these large parasites have evolved with us for millions of years and they have developed ways to deal with it. One of the ways they do this is by dampening down our immune responses—and they do this by secreting compounds that manipulate our immune system. That enables the worms to survive, but it also has benefits for us. The worms are allowed to stay because any serious attempt to kill them would be far too dangerous to the host. So there's an uneasy truce between the worm and us."

Helena agrees with the idea that one of the reasons we have seen this huge rise in allergies and diseases like IBD is that we don't harbor enough Old Friends. What she doesn't approve of is people deliberately self-infecting, as Daniel has done.

"Scientists have worked for over one hundred years to eradicate these diseases and now people want to start reintroducing them? These worms live in the gut and suck blood. They move around. They shed eggs and larvae. If you are infected by too many of them you will become anemic. Yes, we should be finding out how they work, but no, we shouldn't be ordering them up on the internet."

Most scientists would agree with Helena that hookworm simply have too many downsides to be used as medication. Instead, they have been testing more benign parasites, like whipworms. Despite the yuck factor, there have been some successful clinical trials using these worms to treat IBD. In one study[16] they recruited ninety people and infected half with whipworms and gave the others a placebo. None of the volunteers knew which group they were in. Result? Well, 43 percent of patients who got the worms felt better afterward, compared to 17 percent in the placebo group. Not bad, but there's clearly some way to go.

Oddly enough, soon after I met Daniel Hayman I had the opportunity to deliberately infect myself with parasitic worms, in my case rather large ones. I had volunteered to swallow some tapeworm cysts as part of a research project done with scientists from Salford University.

The cysts I swallowed came from a beef tapeworm, *Taenia saginata*, which we got from an abattoir in Kenya. As parasites go, beef tapeworm is relatively harmless and only infects humans and cattle. Pig tapeworm, on the other hand, can be extremely dangerous, as the larvae sometimes migrate to the brain. This is why you should never eat raw or undercooked pork in some of the poorer parts of the world.

There is a widespread belief that tapeworm help you lose weight and in Victorian times it was relatively common for women to swallow tapeworm eggs in the hope of shedding a few pounds. This was almost certainly a waste of time as tapeworm eggs are not infectious to humans. They first have to be eaten by a cow or a bull, where they form a cyst, and it is only if you eat raw, infected meat with cysts in it that you are going to acquire a worm.

But even if you were infected, would you lose weight? I swallowed three tapeworm cysts that we cut out of the tongue of a dead cow (I wanted to be sure I got infected), but despite hosting three worms for a couple of months I actually put on weight.

It could be that the tapeworms were encouraging me to eat more, or it could be that I was unconsciously compensating for them being there. Either way, they didn't seem to be a great weight-loss aid, nor did they create any noticeable problems for me.

In fact, they caused so little trouble that the first time I was absolutely certain that they were really down there was when, two months after swallowing the cysts, I swallowed a pill camera and saw them latched onto the walls of my small intestine, looking very much at home.

Before I started this particular self-experiment I had agreed with my wife that I would kill the tapeworms before they were fully mature. Once they are fully grown they start to shed segments, which crawl around looking for a new host. Understandably my wife was not keen to share our bed with any tapeworm segments which might have come out of me during the night.

One tapeworm expert I know, who deliberately infected himself as part of a research project, had the unpleasant experience of feeling a segment crawl down his trouser leg while driving along the highway.

Anyway, once I had seen and filmed the young tapeworms in my gut, and completed a round of tests, I took some pills and that was the end of the experiment. Although I kept on looking, the worms never came out so I can only assume that, when they had died off, my body treated them just like food and digested them. An ironic end—parasites eaten by their host.

Summary

- Microbes influence our immune system. The "good" ones, our Old Friends, are particularly important when it comes to teaching our immune system how to behave.

- A lack of Old Friends leads to an overactive immune system and an increased risk of allergies.

- As we'll see in a moment, bolstering our Old Friends can help us stay healthy.

5

The Clever Gut Diet

Now we've done a quick tour of the marvelous, murky world of the gut, it's time to have a look at what you can do to keep your gut garden in good shape. In this chapter I will show you how you can improve your biome by changing what you eat and drink. I will also look at what you should avoid.

You are what you feed your biome

These days, when I put something in my mouth, I consider what it will do not just to my body, but also to my biome. Every food decision you make ("Shall I have that slice of cake or that handful of almonds?") decides the fate of countless billions living in your colon. It is quite a responsibility.

Although the following recommendations are based on the latest science, you should take them as guidelines rather than gospel. If you have IBS then you may have to avoid some of the foods we suggest, at least until you have gotten on top of your condition. See Part II, How to Reboot Your Biome, on page 186.

I'm a fan of whole grains, like rye, but they are not going to do you much good if you have a gluten intolerance or celiac disease. And even if you have no gut problems, the response to exactly the same foods varies from person to person. So do experiment with these foods and our recipes, and see which suit you.

Having said all that, there are some foods that are better for you than others. The Clever Gut Diet draws on foods and spices from around the world, including the Mediterranean, India, and Asia. For a diverse gut it is helpful to eat from a range of cuisines.

I'll start with foods most commonly found in my favorite way of eating, the Mediterranean diet. I love Mediterranean food, mainly because it's so tasty, but also because numerous studies have shown that this is an incredibly healthy way to eat.

One of the most impressive dietary studies ever done, the Predimed study, showed that, compared to going on a classic low-fat diet, going on a Mediterranean diet will cut your risk of heart disease, type 2 diabetes, breast cancer, and even stop your brain from shrinking.[17]

For this study, which was funded by the Spanish government, researchers randomly allocated 7,400 overweight Spaniards to either a low-fat diet (lean meat, low-fat dairy, minimal use of oil) or a Mediterranean diet (oily nuts, oily fish, lots of olive oil, eggs, dark chocolate, red wine). They were then followed for many years. The results were clear.

Although they were not calorie restricted, those randomized to the Mediterranean diet put on less weight, particularly around the middle, than those on the low-fat diet. They were 30 percent less likely to develop heart disease and half as likely to develop type 2 diabetes. A particularly important element of the diet seemed to be olive oil. In fact, women in this study who were asked to add an extra couple of teaspoons of extra-virgin olive oil a day cut their risk of developing breast cancer by nearly 68 percent, compared to those who were dutifully eating low fat.

Foods that nourish the gut

Olive oil

As well as adding flavor and taste, olive oil is one of the healthiest fats you can eat because it's rich in a range of polyphenols and antioxidants, which are good at damping down inflammation, whether in the brain, the breast, or the gut.

Olive oil is one of those good fats that fills you up, so you'll be less tempted to eat processed fat and sugar later in the day.

Should you buy ordinary or extra-virgin olive oil? For me it comes down to cost, convenience, and personal taste. I cook with the ordinary (contrary to popular myth, olive oil is one of the most stable oils you can fry with) and splash the extra-virgin on my salads.

103

Be aware, however, that not all extra-virgin is extra virgin. Because it is expensive to produce, extra-virgin olive oil is now one of the two most counterfeited foods in the world (Manuka honey is the other).

The counterfeiting has been going on for many years, but the scandal erupted in 2010 when researchers at the University of California, Davis, tested a wide range of imported extra-virgin olive oils, mainly from Italy. More than 70 percent of the oils failed their tests either because they were rancid or had been adulterated by other, cheaper oils.

According to Tom Mueller, a journalist and author of *Extra Virginity: The Sublime and Scandalous World of Olive Oil*, this is a widespread problem, particularly in Italy, where it involves the Mafia and other crime syndicates. Popular ways to adulterate extra-virgin olive oil include adding canola oil or much poorer-quality olive oils. The blended oil is then chemically deodorized and sold as extra-virgin oil.

Unless you have access to a well-equipped laboratory, there is no reliable way of detecting this adulteration. There are lots of urban myths about testing olive oil, such as putting it in the fridge to see if it solidifies, or trying to light it and seeing how it burns. None of these home-based tests work. If you want to find out more about which brands you can trust, and which you can't, visit my website clever guts .com, as this is a field that is evolving all the time.

Oily fish

Like olive oil, oily fish are full of good fats, which are anti-inflammatory. In the case of oily fish, the key ingredient is omega-3. Unfortunately, white fish, like cod, don't contain many omega-3 fatty acids and they don't provide anything like the same health benefits. That said, even nonoily fish are a good source of protein. Not long ago "experts" were worried about oily fish because of its high fat content and you still see some government websites recommending the nonoily versions.

One of my favorite maverick self-experimenters, Professor Hugh Sinclair of Oxford University, helped set the record straight.

In the 1940s Hugh Sinclair traveled to northern Canada to study the people living in the Arctic. Once known as Eskimos, they are now officially called the Inuit.

During his stay Hugh became intrigued by the fact that, although the Inuit ate lots of fat and very few vegetables, they had relatively low rates of heart disease.

He did further research and concluded that omega-3—an essential fatty acid found abundantly in oily fish—was protecting the Inuit from heart attacks. He wrote a number of articles about this, but was largely ignored. So in 1979 he decided to put himself on an Inuit diet, consisting of seal, oily fish, mollusks, and crustaceans.

He suspected, based on animal studies, that eating lots of fish oils would, at the very least, increase his clotting time. As the name implies, "clotting time" is a measure of how long it takes your blood to clot. This is important in heart disease because it is the forming of a blood clot, which breaks off and blocks one of your arteries that ultimately leads to a heart attack or stroke.

A few years ago I decided to repeat his experiment myself, though I had to skip eating seal (I ordered some from Canada but it got impounded in customs). I also couldn't stomach the idea of fish with every meal so I confined myself to one portion of oily fish a day. Hugh Sinclair was on his diet for three months; I managed one month.

Like him, before I started on my fishy diet I did some tests, which included measuring my clotting time. Over the course of the month I repeated the tests a number of times.

By the end of the experiment my "bad" cholesterol levels had halved and my clotting time had doubled. Hugh Sinclair, on his more extreme diet, saw his clotting time go up from three minutes to a frankly terrifying fifty minutes. I say terrifying because if you have an injury and start to bleed it is useful to be able to clot, otherwise you risk bleeding to death.

To cut a long story short, it is now widely accepted that eating oily fish at least twice a week reduces not only the risk of heart disease but also anxiety, depression, and inflammatory conditions such as arthritis. But what effect does it have on your biome?

Well, following in the footsteps of the great Hugh Sinclair, a human volunteer recently offered himself up as a guinea pig for trial by fish.[18]

The subject, who is just described in the study as a

"forty-five-year-old Caucasian male," had a reasonable diet before he started, which included red meat and vegetables. For a couple of weeks he changed to a fish-protein-only diet, which added up to just over 600 mg (less than an ounce) of omega-3 a day.

During the course of his new diet, the researchers, naturally enough, took lots of stool samples. They saw what they described as a "remarkable increase" in the levels of a number of bacteria associated with butyrate production. As I've pointed out before, butyrate plays a key role in maintaining gut health. It is the major source of energy for your colonic mucosa (the mucous lining that protects your colon) and it also helps reduce inflammation.

He then reverted to his normal diet. Unfortunately, after a couple of fish-free weeks, his stool samples returned to where they had been before. It seems that if you want to keep the benefits you have to keep eating the fish.

Good examples of oily fish include salmon, tuna, trout, sardines, mackerel, and herring. Some people are anxious about the mercury found in fish, though I think the benefits clearly outweigh the risk. As a precaution, pregnant women are advised to limit the amount of high-mercury fish they eat.

You can get more details about levels of mercury found in different fish from the US government's Food and Drug Administration website.[19]

Below are some average mercury levels, measured in parts per million. As you can see the fish to avoid are swordfish and shark (sharks are, anyway, horribly overfished):

Swordfish: 0.995 ppm
Shark: 0.979 ppm
Canned tuna: 0.128 ppm
Cod: 0.111 ppm
Trout: 0.071 ppm
Mackerel: 0.050 ppm
Salmon: 0.022 ppm
Anchovies: 0.017 ppm
Sardines: 0.013 ppm
Shrimp: 0.001 ppm

You can get omega-3 fatty acids from other foods, such as grass-fed beef, walnuts, flaxseeds, and hemp oil, but they come in a less biologically effective form. Lots of manufactured foods are now being fortified with omega-3, but because the omega-3 they use is extracted from algae it has a fishy aroma. Since potential customers would, understandably, be put off by things like fishy-smelling margarine, manufacturers mask the smell chemically. The resulting food is unlikely to be as healthy as you would hope.

As well as fish, an excellent natural source of omega-3 is seaweed (see page 132).

Fish oil capsules

What happens if you don't like oily fish? Well, there are always fish oil capsules. These are hugely popular but not hugely effective, at least not in humans. Most experts I've talked to are skeptical, and that's because the science doesn't support the claimed health benefits. A large meta-analysis of 89 studies published in 2006 showed no benefit from consuming fish oil capsules, and a more recent study from 2012 published in the *Journal of the American Medical Association*, covering 20 studies and 68,680 patients, also found that taking fish oil capsules made no difference to your chance of having a heart attack or stroke.[20]

Part of the problem may be the poor quality of some fish oil capsules. A research team from New Zealand examined fish oil capsules from all over the world and found that most contained fish oils that were oxidized—i.e., rancid. This was despite them being well within the sell-by date. "Fish oil capsules" sounds wholesome, but it can take three years to get oils from the fish to those plastic bottles you see on pharmacy and supermarket shelves. Omega-3 is relatively unstable and in that time it may go off. Just as eating rancid fish is unlikely to do you much good, swallowing oxidized fish oil is unlikely to lead to a healthy biome.

The best way to tell if a fish oil is off is by taste and smell. If you get an unpleasant fishy burp after consuming a capsule you may have an off pack. Do buy something with a trademark and keep the capsules in the fridge. Or you could just stop taking them altogether, as millions have.

As the *Washington Post* recently put it: "Fish oil pills: A $1.2 billion industry built, so far, on empty promises."

With all this bad publicity it's not surprising that the bottom is dropping out of the lucrative fish oil market, with sales falling internationally. If you really, really don't like fish, I would recommend cod liver oil. Cod liver oil is also an excellent source of vitamin D. I used to hate fish, but I have been converted. We have some fish recipes in this book that I hope will help change your mind.

Meat

So, oily fish is definitely on the menu, but what about meat, particularly red meat, like beef, lamb, and pork? In recent years I've seen plenty of headlines along the lines of "All red meat is risky," and "If you want to live longer, hold the red meat."

Really? On the plus side we know that red meat is a great source of protein. Beef, whole or ground, is also an excellent source of iron and vitamin B_{12}, which are vital for producing healthy blood cells, and in which many people are chronically deficient. What's more, vitamin B_{12} is an essential nutrient for the developing brain, one of my favorite organs.

On the not-so-plus side, red meat is also rich in saturated fat. Beef has about nine times more saturated fat per gram than tofu. But is saturated fat as bad as is often claimed?

I recently met up with Dr. Ronald Krauss, one of the world's most respected nutrition researchers. Dr. Krauss is based at the Children's Hospital Oakland Research Institute in California. He has spent his professional life investigating the link between saturated fat and heart disease. He has very personal reasons for doing so.

"My father had a heart attack when I was very young," he told me. "This had such an impact on me that I decided when I was six years old that I was going to try and do something about heart disease."

He trained as a doctor, then immersed himself in research. Because of his family history, he was concerned about his own health, so naturally he followed the dietary advice of the time, going on a low-fat diet and shunning cholesterol-rich eggs.

He also put his patients and research subjects on this diet. The trouble was, it didn't produce the results that they were expecting. "We thought that everybody would get better on this diet, that their cholesterol profile would improve. In many cases they got worse."

The problem was that when you go on a low-fat diet you

have to eat something else. The "something else" was often carbohydrates, like bread, pasta, or potatoes.

Dr. Krauss discovered that eating carbohydrates increases levels of a particularly damaging form of cholesterol known as small particle LDL (low-density lipoprotein).

Yet most doctors believed that saturated fat was the enemy. So with colleagues he decided to do a meta-analysis, pulling together as many high-quality studies as they could find. When, in 2010, they published their findings in the *American Journal of Clinical Nutrition*,[21] it was a bombshell. "We found the heart attack risk was slightly higher but not significant. Stroke risk was actually reduced. So overall if you took it across the entire range of disease, heart disease and stroke, there was absolutely zero effect."

Other more recent meta-analyses, such as one from Cambridge University, funded by the British Heart Foundation,[22] came to similar conclusions.

Dr. Krauss doesn't see any harm in eating red meat a couple of days a week, although he prefers fish, topped up with vegetables and nuts. "I stay away from potatoes as much as possible but my real weakness is bread. I have half a bagel most days, because I cannot resist them. Sugar almost never except for a little dessert with some chocolate. My main indulgence is a small piece after dinner because I consider chocolate an essential nutrient."

Other American experts, like Dr. Walter Willett, who is based at the Harvard T. H. Chan School of Public Health, are less enthusiastic about red meat.

"In our studies we've shown that those who consumed higher amounts of red meat had a higher risk of total mortality, cardiovascular mortality, and cancer mortality," he told me in the Harvard cafeteria, while I nonchalantly ate a steak. Dr. Willett almost never eats meat.

According to Dr. Willett, eating 85 grams (3 ounces) a day—a small steak—increases your risk of premature death by 13 percent.

This surprised me because a massive European study,[23] has come to exactly the opposite conclusion. In this study, which involved following nearly half a million people in ten European countries for over twelve years, scientists found that eating moderate amounts of red meat had no effect on mortality.

If anything, it seemed to be protective. If you ate over 160 grams (5½ ounces) of red meat a day, then, yes, you were at greater risk of heart disease and cancer. But those eating less were no worse off than nonmeat eaters, and possibly a little healthier.

So how do you explain all these apparently conflicting studies? Well, one of the things that struck me was that the European study was done in Europe, where farmers are not allowed to routinely feed antibiotics and growth promoters to animals. In the US (where Dr. Willett's studies are based) things are very different.

If you have ever visited one of those huge industrial cattle factories down in Texas, as I have, and watched the cattle being fed corn, antibiotics, growth promoters, and a bit of green dye (to make the whole thing look more palatable), then you might not be surprised that Americans eating this sort of meat don't do too well.

I think what's important is not so much whether the meat you are eating is red or not, but what that meat itself has been reared on. If it has been brought up on antibiotics and growth promoters, it is unlikely to be doing you or your biome any good.

I continue to eat red meat, good quality and grass-fed, once or twice a week. But before carnivores go off rejoicing, I have to tell you that processed meat (like bacon, ham, sausages, and salami) is quite a different story. More on that on page 156.

Three other foods that have been demonized but which are surprisingly good for your gut

Cocoa

Whoever invented milk chocolate was an evil genius. It is the most craved food on the planet. I have tried to give it up on many occasions and failed miserably. My kids know that if they leave chocolate anywhere visible around the house, I will probably eat it. I no longer buy milk chocolate because I know that once I start on a bar I simply will not stop. A few weeks ago I was driving home, alone, and stopped to buy some gas. While I was there I "accidentally" found myself buying a bar of milk chocolate. When I returned to the car I threw the bar of chocolate into the back, hoping to remove temptation. Instead, I thought about that chocolate for the next ten miles and eventually had to pull over to eat it.

There are a number of reasons why milk chocolate is so seductive, including the flavor, smell, and the way it melts in your mouth. And, of course, the marketing. But what it also has is the magic 50:50 ratio. Half of the calories in a bar of chocolate come from sugar, half from fat. You will find the same is true of a lot of the foods you crave, including doughnuts and ice cream.

Although we talk about sugar being "addictive," few of us would eat a bowl of sugar by itself. Similarly, few of us would drink a glass of cream. But mix them together, add some flavorings, freeze, and you have ice cream, which is impossibly tantalizing.

Why is this 50:50 ratio so important? Well, perhaps because it was there in the first food you ever consumed. Breast milk has a 50:50 ratio of calories from sugar to calories from fat which you will find nowhere else in the unprocessed foods you eat. Melon is high in sugar, but not fat. Steak has lots of fat, but no sugar. It is one of those theories that would be hard to prove but certainly sounds plausible to me.

Whatever the reason, I am hopelessly hooked on chocolate. To overcome these cravings, my main strategy has been to switch to eating dark chocolate, which has less sugar and which I find far less addictive. I'm also pleased to say that dark chocolate is one of the things that the Mediterranean diet says is fine to eat, particularly if it has a high cocoa content. The problem with chocolate, health-wise, is not the cocoa, but the sugar. Cocoa itself is surprisingly good for you. It is broken down in your colon to produce nitric oxide, which expands your arteries and is good for your cardiovascular system. Cocoa is also an excellent source of flavonoids and polyphenols which, as we've seen, are good for your gut bacteria.

Eggs

I eat eggs most mornings. Not so long ago this was considered nutritional suicide. Like fat, cholesterol was demonized. If it was common sense that fat would clog up your arteries, then it was obvious that foods rich in cholesterol, like eggs and seafood, would do the same. We were urged to eat no more than a couple of eggs a week and lots of people started eating egg-white-only omelets, which was a terrible shame because almost all the nutrients are in the yolk.

Well, it turns out that like the fear of fat, the fear of eggs was also totally misplaced. A meta-analysis of seventeen studies published in the *British Medical Journal* concluded that "higher consumption of eggs is not associated with increased risk of coronary heart disease or stroke."[24] Government guidelines around the world have now done a complete about-face, and we're all being encouraged to eat more eggs.

Whether scrambled, boiled, poached, or in an omelet, eggs are a superb source of protein, rich in vitamins and minerals. There are around 90 calories in a boiled egg, half those in a small bowl of Frosted Flakes with milk and a quarter of those in a croissant with butter and jam (400 calories, plus). Unlike the cereal or the croissant, the protein in the eggs will keep you feeling fuller for longer.

I can't find any studies which show that eating eggs will do great things to your biome, but if it stops you having sugary cereal for breakfast or scarfing down that muffin mid-morning, then that is mission accomplished.

Wine

We all know that large amounts of alcohol are very bad for us, but what about more modest quantities? In the famous Predimed study, the volunteers who were randomized to the Mediterranean diet were allowed a glass or two of wine with their evening meal. Yet this flies in the face of much current medical advice, which states that any amount of alcohol is likely to do harm. So where does the truth lie?

A recent study in the US[25] supports the claim that modest amounts of alcohol can be healthy. In this study they followed more than 14,000 adults aged forty-five and older for twenty-four years. What they found is that those who drank up to twelve units of alcohol per week (the equivalent of around six glasses of wine a week) had a lower risk of developing heart failure than those who never drank alcohol. But what about the biome?

Now, on the face of it, your microbiome should really hate alcohol. Pure alcohol is death to anything that is microscopic. That's why we use alcohol-infused swabs if we really want to clean our hands. We also know that alcohol can inflame the stomach, which is not a good thing. But alcoholic drinks like wine contain more than just alcohol. They also contain polyphenols.

As we've seen, polyphenols are chemicals found in tea, coffee, wine, fruit, vegetables, and chocolate. When you eat these foods, around half of what you consume passes straight through the small intestine to the large intestine, where it has a powerful influence on the microbiome.

To see exactly what effect the polyphenols in red wine are having, Spanish researchers recruited ten healthy middle-aged men and asked them to take part in an experiment.[26] After an alcohol-free week they were randomly allocated to drinking either a large glass of red wine (270 ml or 1 generous cup), red wine with the alcohol removed, or gin (100 ml or about ½ cup) each day with their evening meal. After twenty days they switched regimens—each volunteer had to follow all three of them. Throughout this experiment blood samples and stool samples were taken on a regular basis.

What the researchers found was that when the volunteers were drinking the red wine, and to a lesser extent when they drank de-alcoholized wine, there were significant drops in blood pressure, in C-reactive protein (CRP—a measure of inflammation), and in their triglyceride levels (the amount of fat circulating in the blood).

In addition, there was a marked change in their gut bacteria, with a particular increase in *Bacteroidetes*, the type of bacteria associated with slimness. They also noticed a significant increase in *Bifidobacteria*, which are associated with lowering cholesterol.

When it comes to booze, red wine seems to trump white wine, while spirits offer no obvious health benefits. As for beer, which is also known as "liquid toast," I tend to avoid it because of its high carbohydrate content. If you are trying to lose weight or if you have sulfur-reducing bacteria in your gut, then beer is definitely a no-no.

Fruit and vegetables

Everyone knows that fruit and vegetables are good for us, but even those who manage to cram in their five a day or more, tend to stick to an incredibly limited range of them. Although most of us have realized that there is life beyond carrots, lettuces, and tomatoes, we are not particularly adventurous in our eating habits. And that means our biome ends up being pretty limited as well. One simple way to increase your variety is to introduce more color to your plate (remember Dave, with the IBS, and his beige diet? That, I'm sorry to say, is a very common cause of gut problems).

Apart from the fact that it makes your meal look more appealing, why should you go for color? Well, the pigments that plants produce not only give them their color but also keep them healthy, as they are made up of hundreds of different bioactive compounds or phytonutrients. Eating a wide variety of different colored fruits and vegetables will give your gut bacteria something to chew on, as well as providing nutrients.

Phytonutrients

Phytonutrients, also known as phytochemicals, are concentrated in the skins of fruits and vegetables and are responsible for their color, scent, and flavor. They also help protect the plant from fungi and bacteria. The best-known phytonutrients are carotenoids, flavonoids, and polyphenols. Carotenoids and flavonoids are found in yellow, orange, red, blue, and purple fruits and vegetables (see the Phyto Salad recipe, page 223). Polyphenols are found in foods like cocoa, olives, dark chocolate, tea, coffee, and red wine. Dried herbs are also spectacularly rich in them.[27]

Green

There are two types of green vegetable. Leafy greens, such as spinach, chard, lettuce, and kale, are a good source of essential minerals, including magnesium, manganese, and potassium. Spinach is also rich in folate and betaine, which help regulate homocysteine (high levels of which are associated with heart disease).

The other major class of green vegetables is the brassicas, which contain sulfur and organosulfur compounds. These include cabbage, cauliflower, and broccoli. Sulfur is essential for the production of glutathione, an important antioxidant, as well as amino acids that are essential for building tissue and muscle.

But a word of warning: if you have IBD you may do well to avoid them. Although sulfur is great for healthy guts, it can aggravate inflamed ones.

There is a significant social downside to eating sulphur-rich foods, too. Even people with a normal gut sometimes find that eating members of the brassica family (particularly brussels sprouts) can lead to awful smells. That's because a third of the population have high levels of sulfate-reducing bacteria in their guts, which turn the sulfur in their diet into hydrogen sulfide (which produces the smell of rotten eggs). If you evacuate a room after you've eaten a brassica or had a few pints of beer and a white bread sandwich (both of which also contain a lot of sulfur), you know why.

Yellow, orange, and red: carotenoids

Fruit and vegetables that are orange, yellow, or red are often rich in carotenoids. Carotenoids also give autumn leaves their vibrant colors. Foods rich in carotenoids include, not surprisingly, carrots. The type of carotenoid you find in carrots can be converted to retinol, an active form of vitamin A. The fact that vitamin A is important for healthy eyesight may explain why carrots are supposed to help you see in the dark. But you also find carotenoids in egg yolks, bananas, melons, tomatoes, peppers, and squash. One particularly popular, carotene-rich fruit is the tomato. Thanks to its intense umami flavor, the tomato is the most popular fruit in the world. And no, it's not a vegetable.

Black, green, yellow: flavonoids

The word flavonoid comes from the Latin word flavus meaning yellow, and in a plant, this versatile substance not only attracts insects for pollination but also helps protect it from harmful ultraviolet light. In humans, flavonoids may help combat allergies, inflammation, and infection, as well as the consequences of yo-yo dieting. Despite the original meaning of the name, foods that have a high flavonoid content come in a range of colors and include parsley, black tea, red wine, apples, cocoa, and peanuts.

Blue and purple

Blue and purple foods get their coloring from a type of flavonoid called anthocyanins. The more intense the color, the greater the concentration of anthocyanins. You'll find high levels of these particular flavonoids in blackberries, blueberries, purple carrots, red cabbage, and the skin of eggplant.

Eating anthocyanin-rich blueberries may improve memory as we get older. They also strongly encourage the growth of "good" bacteria such as *Bifidobacterium* and *Lactobacillus*.

White

Examples of phytonutrient-rich white foods include garlic, white onions, shallots, and leeks. These are rich in alliums and allyl sulfur compounds. The most intensely studied of this particular group is garlic, which has been used down the centuries for medical reasons, as well as in cooking.

Although there is no compelling evidence that garlic will ward off vampires, it does appear to be quite good at killing "bad" microbes. Traditionally it was eaten raw to treat coughs, colds, and croup. A clinical trial, using a garlic infusion as a mouthwash, showed positive results, although the ensuing garlic breath was a significant drawback.

Herbs and spices

Many dried herbs like thyme, oregano, and basil are rich in polyphenols, while ginger and cumin have anti-inflammatory effects. But the spice with the greatest reputation for being gut-friendly is turmeric.

Turmeric
Turmeric is a yellowy-orange spice that is very popular in South Asian cooking. It gives a distinctive color to dishes like chicken tikka masala and curried cauliflower soup. Multiple health claims have been made about turmeric. But do they stand up?

There are at least two hundred different compounds in turmeric, but the one that's of particular interest to scientists is called curcumin. A recent review article looking at the evidence[28] concluded that turmeric has powerful antioxidant and anti-inflammatory properties. It is good at inhibiting the growth of "bad" bacteria, parasites, and pathogenic fungi, and it directly protects the wall of the intestine.

Most human studies have been done with high doses of turmeric or curcumin taken in capsule form. But how well does it work when taken in food? Recently, I was involved in an experiment in which we randomly allocated a group of nearly one hundred volunteers to either a teaspoon of turmeric every day, a placebo, or a supplement. Those who got the turmeric cooked with it, added it to soup, sprinkled it on yogurt, or stirred it into warm milk. Not everyone was crazy about the flavor. "Strong and lingering" was how some people described it.

Nonetheless, they stuck with it and after just six weeks we saw some significant changes in the activity of a number of genes in the turmeric-consuming group.

Professor Martin Widschwendter from University College, London, who ran the experiment, was surprised and delighted by the results. "It was really exciting, to be honest," he told me. "We found one particular gene which showed the biggest difference. And what's interesting is that we know this particular gene is involved in three specific diseases: depression, asthma, and eczema, and cancer. This is a really striking finding."

A lot more research needs to be done, but I think turmeric is a spice that's well worth using. We have included it in a number of our recipes, including a delicious latte (see page 205). You will find that adding pepper increases its bioavailability—the amount of the active compound your gut absorbs. I like a sprinkle of turmeric with a touch of red pepper flakes and pepper in an omelet in the morning.

Fiber

Eating more fruit and vegetables also means you are going to be getting more fiber, which is normally a good thing as most of us don't eat enough. In a typical Western diet, we consume less than half the recommended amount, which is at least 25 grams (about 1 ounce) a day.

For most people, boosting fiber intake is likely to be good for the guts, the heart, and the waistline. But if you have a diseased gut, adding more fiber to your diet may actually make you feel worse.

Prebiotics—treats for the Old Friends

Although fiber in almost any form is helpful, there are some types that are particularly important when it comes to keeping your gut bacteria in good shape. These are known as "prebiotics." A prebiotic is a special type of plant fiber which your body can't digest but which encourages the growth of "good" bacteria in your gut. The "good" gut bacteria turn that prebiotic fiber into chemicals like butyrate. As I mentioned before, butyrate has been shown to have powerful anti-inflammatory effects inside the bowel. Prebiotics act a bit like a fertilizer, boosting the growth of "good" bacteria.

Inulin

This is one of the best known of the prebiotics. It is found in lots of different plants, but in high concentrations in only a few. As well as promoting a healthier biome and reducing constipation, eating food with lots of inulin in it can improve your bone health, as it enhances calcium absorption, and reduce your risk of heart disease, as it lowers blood triglyceride levels. Foods rich in inulin include:

1. *Onions, leeks, and garlic*

Yes, it's them again. They are packed with inulin. Fortunately, I love this particular family of plants and cook with them on a regular basis. Our recipes are full of them. The Spanish make a wonderful tomato base called *sofrito*, which consists of garlic, onion, paprika, and tomatoes all cooked together in olive oil. It's delicious with chicken, fish, or shrimp. A treat for your family and your biome. We have a tomato sauce recipe in the back (see page 254).

2. *Chicory*

Chicory is normally eaten in salad. It has pale, slightly bitter leaves tinged with green or purple. This group also includes radicchio with its variegated red and white leaves. It is a member of the sunflower and daisy family, a close relative of lettuce and dandelions. In some countries chicory leaves are still crushed and used as a poultice to treat skin inflammations. The root is particularly rich in inulin—it accounts for nearly half its fiber. You are most likely to encounter chicory root as a caffeine-free coffee substitute.

3. Dandelion greens

These are good in salads and a great source of inulin. To make the leaves more palatable, you can blanch them to remove the bitterness or sauté them like spinach. They are less bitter before the flower head appears. Adding a handful to a salad gives it extra flavor and crunch. You don't have to go far to find them as they grow as a weed. You can also buy them from health food stores. Dandelions are used in traditional herbal medicine to treat infections and liver problems (you can make a bitter enzyme-inducing salad from a few simple ingredients, as listed on page 212).

4. Jerusalem artichoke

Over 70 percent of the Jerusalem artichoke's fiber comes from inulin, so as much as 1 to 2 percent of its weight is inulin, making it one of the richest sources of this prebiotic. It is also known as "sunchoke" in the US or "fartichoke" because the high levels of non-digestible carbohydrate almost inevitably lead to some flatulence. If you are dining on them, leave the window open. If you aren't a regular vegetable eater or you have IBS, Jerusalem artichokes are probably one to avoid. We include a delicious Jerusalem artichoke soup in the recipe section (see page 218). In addition to inulin, Jerusalem artichokes provide lots of vitamin B$_1$, iron, potassium, and a decent amount of copper and vitamin C.

5. *Asparagus*

As well as being almost 3 percent inulin, asparagus is surprisingly rich in protein. I like to steam it for a few minutes, then flash-cook it over a grill and eat it hot with lemon juice and butter. The only downside of eating asparagus is that a few hours later you may produce strange-smelling urine. Speaking from personal experience, it has a distinct hint of sulfur, which can take you by surprise if you are not expecting it. Not everyone produces a strong smell in their urine after eating asparagus and not everyone can detect it.

There is a statistic for almost everything—studies in the UK and the US have come up with different figures for the percentage of the population who produce strange smells after eating asparagus. A British study from 1987[29] found that only 43 percent of British males produce an obvious smell after eating asparagus, and it runs in families. A US study[30] found that 79 percent of Americans produced a detectable odor.

6. *Bananas*

Bananas contain modest amounts of inulin, less than 1 percent of their weight, but they are rich in a number of minerals and vitamins, though they also include a fair amount of sugar. It's particularly worth including green or unripe bananas in your diet because they are a good source of resistant starch, which is another very important prebiotic.

Resistant starch (RS)

Resistant starch is a type of starch that, as its name implies, resists digestion in your stomach and small intestine and reaches your colon largely intact. You are unlikely to get big blood sugar spikes after eating RS, and you won't hold on to many calories from it either. Once it reaches the large intestine, it feeds the "good" bacteria which digest it and release butyrate. As we've already seen, butyrate reduces inflammation and strengthens the gut wall.

You'll find lots of resistant starch in grains, seeds, and legumes. You also get it in unripe bananas and green peas. But one of the more surprising places you will find some of it is in pasta or rice that has been cooked and cooled.

I first became aware of this curious finding when researchers from a program I worked on asked Dr. Denise Robertson, from the University of Surrey, to run a slightly odd experiment. Volunteers were asked to eat pasta with a tomato sauce either hot, cold, or reheated. Their blood sugar levels were measured after each meal and we discovered, as we'd expected, that eating cold pasta led to a smaller spike in blood glucose and insulin than eating freshly boiled pasta. That's because cooking and cooling pasta changes the structure of the starch in the pasta, making it more resistant to digestion.

But then we found something that we didn't expect—

cooking, cooling, and reheating the pasta had an even more dramatic effect. Or, to be precise, eating reheated pasta resulted in an even smaller effect on blood sugar levels than eating cooled pasta. In our volunteers it reduced the rise in blood sugar levels by 50 percent. This strongly suggests that reheating the pasta made it into an even more resistant starch. As far as I know it's something that had never been measured before.

Since we ran that experiment, a group in Sri Lanka has done something similar with rice. They found that if they boiled rice with a bit of coconut oil, cooled it down, then reheated it in a microwave, they could increase the levels of resistant starch in it roughly fifteen-fold. They think that eating rice this way probably halves the amount of calories your gut will absorb from it.

At the very least it is a good excuse to use up any leftover pasta or rice you may have in the fridge. And by the way, the claim that reheating rice is dangerous is an almost total myth. Unless it has been sitting out in a warm place for many hours it should be absolutely fine.

For a list of foods with the most resistant starch, see page 268.

Other good sources of fiber

Barley

Barley is an ancient and very tasty grain with a slightly nutty flavor. It is good in soups and stews, really giving them a bite. Barley scores well as a prebiotic because it contains lots of beta-glucan. Like inulin, beta-glucan promotes the growth of friendly bacteria in your gut. Beta-glucan binds LDL or "bad" cholesterol in your gut, preventing it from being absorbed through the wall lining, thereby lowering levels in the blood.

Oats

Like barley, whole oats contain large amounts of beta-glucan fiber, as well as some resistant starch. I did a small experiment, in which I ate oats every morning for a month and discovered that it cut my "bad" cholesterol by about 10 percent. Using whole oats, the sort of porridge that takes longer to cook, will also slow the release of the starchy carbohydrates and sugars, and the fiber is more likely to get to feed the good guys in your biome, whereas more processed, quick-cook porridge is less filling and will produce a greater sugar spike. (See our granola recipe on page 198.)

Flaxseed

This is another very healthy prebiotic, a seed with a slightly nutty flavor. You can scatter flaxseed on your porridge in the morning, or try adding it toasted to salads for a delicious crunch. Flaxseed is a reasonable source of omega-3 though, unlike fish, little of it is in an active form that your body can make use of. It is, however, rich in insoluble fiber, like cellulose. As well as feeding your microbiome, the fiber in flaxseed should ensure regular bowel movements. (See our recipe for Green Flaxseed Bread on page 210.)

Apples

I love apples and they are one of the healthiest fruits you can eat, as long as you consume them whole and not as a juice. They are another good prebiotic, low in sugar and high in pectin. Eating apples increases the production of our Old Friend butyrate, the short-chain fatty acid that feeds our "good" bacteria. They are also high in polyphenol antioxidants. I love stewed apples with yogurt, or diced and cooked in the oven with a scattering of cinnamon (see page 260).

Seaweed

Slippery, slimy, and with a very distinctive ocean flavor, seaweed is not something I'd had much experience of before researching this book. It is a popular food in many parts of the world, particularly Japan, China, Korea, and Taiwan. Seaweed comes in a wide range of colors including green, brown, and red. Modern land plants are all derived from the green species of seaweed, which gives you some idea of just how diverse these sea plants are.

The seaweed species you are most likely to have encountered on your plate is nori, which is used to make sushi. Other common types include dulse, which I was told tastes like bacon when fried—it doesn't; kelp, which is used as a gluten-free alternative to noodles; and spirulina.

Not all seaweeds are edible, and some are poisonous, so unless you know what you are doing it is not a great idea to pluck it from the seashore and wolf it down.

But the seaweeds that are edible are excellent prebiotics, packed with vitamins and minerals, as well as fiber and omega-3 fatty acids. With all this going for them it's not surprising that they have been hailed as yet another superfood. But where's the evidence?

Well, there have been lots of animal studies that have suggested benefits. Researchers from University College, Dublin, for example, have shown that feeding seaweed extract to sows produces long-lasting effects on their offspring. Their piglets have less of the nasty bacteria, such as *E. coli*, in the gut; they need fewer antibiotics during their lifetime; and they put on weight far faster than piglets fed on a standard diet. But what about human studies?

Dr. Pia Winberg, who works at the University of Wollongong in Australia, describes herself as a seaweed farmer. She is incredibly enthusiastic about the potential of seaweed, pointing out its long history: "Seaweed is one of the oldest 'plants' used by humans and records reach back to Tasmanian aboriginal communities." People have been eating seaweed for thousands of years.

She also says that you will find seaweed in toothpaste, paint, printer ink, ice cream, and salad dressing. Scientists are even testing seaweed gel nasal spray products against bird flu. But it's the impact of seaweed on the microbiome that really interests her, something she has been assessing not just in the lab but at home.

"I've done lots of tests on my kids and everyone else I can lay my hands on. Blood, urine, and feces are always exciting for kids."

She has just completed one of the first human trials on

the effects of seaweed on the gut, which she plans to publish in 2017. For her study she recruited sixty-four people who were either overweight or obese. They were then randomly allocated to consume one of three capsules every day for six weeks. One of the capsules contained 2 grams (0.07 ounces) of a special seaweed fiber, the second capsule contained 4 grams (0.141 ounces), and the final capsule was a placebo.

The volunteers went away and swallowed a capsule every day for six weeks, with neither they nor the scientists knowing who was consuming seaweed and who was getting the placebo. Blood and stool samples were taken at the beginning of the study and then again at the end. So what did they discover?

"What we found," Pia told me, "was a significant reduction in inflammation and an increase in insulin sensitivity. What we also found, when we looked at their stool, was that a group of about fifteen different bacteria had increased in the people who were on the active seaweed supplements."

These bacteria were mainly from groups which produce short-chain fatty acids like butyrate, which in turn encourage the growth of the mucous lining.

But what Pia found particularly interesting were some of the other benefits.

"Thanks to the increased fiber, everyone taking the seaweed supplements reported becoming more regular. I hadn't appreciated before the study how many people are constipated. At the end of the trial, when they found out what they had been consuming, people wanted to keep on taking the capsules, just for that reason."

The volunteers taking the seaweed capsules also reported feeling less desire for sugar and fast carbs, which Pia thinks may be because the seaweed had changed their gut flora. This in turn could explain the improvements she saw in their insulin levels.

"Did the seaweed make any of them gassy?" I asked.

"We didn't find that in this study," Pia replied. "In fact a couple of participants with IBS reported that for the first time they could eat cabbage and other brassica-type vegetables. That is anecdotal but interesting.

"The most surprising and stunning result," she went on, "was with a woman who had severe psoriasis. It was so bad on her hands that the skin just constantly flaked off. She had been in bandages for two years and lost her job. Four weeks into the study she took the bandages off and her skin looked fine. At the end of the study she stopped taking the capsules. Three weeks later her hands started peeling again.

"When she was taking the capsule the inflammatory factors in her blood went down, so it seems likely that the reduced inflammation was helping her skin. We've tested her five times now, putting her on and off the seaweed, and each time she is off her hands peel. When she goes back on the psoriasis ends." Pia and her team are now extending their clinical studies, looking specifically at people with psoriatic skin disorders.

The main downside to seaweed is that it has a fishy taste. Nonetheless, we have included a number of recipes in this book that have been tested on some very picky consumers, including my children, and had the thumbs-up. If you want to find out more about Pia's work and how to buy capsules containing seaweed dietary fiber, visit our website. When Pia publishes her study, we will post a link to it.

Probiotics—how to introduce more Old Friends

Unlike prebiotics, which are like fertilizers for your biome, probiotics are the live bacteria or yeast that you parachute into your intestine, in the hope that they will take root and do you some good.

To have a chance of reaching your colon alive, probiotics first have to survive a dunking in the acid bath of your stomach, followed by a dousing in gastric juices and a lot of pounding along the way. Even if they reach the colon they still face a vast army of microbes that are already in residence and unlikely to welcome any newcomers.

There's a lot of hype around probiotics, with lots of different supplements being advertised on the internet and in health food stores. Only a few have decent science behind them, and I will come to those in a moment. Unless you have a particular gut condition you are trying to treat (like antibiotic-induced diarrhea), I think the best way to top up your levels of "good" bacteria is through food. And one of the best probiotic foods is homemade yogurt.

Yogurt

I've made yogurt many times—it is so much nicer than the store-bought stuff, as well being richer in bacteria like *Lactobacillus* (see our recipe on page 206).

When I buy yogurt it is usually live and full-fat. I add fruits to sweeten it, or scatter cinnamon, flaxseed, and nuts over it. The sugary low-fat versions are unlikely to have any health-promoting properties. The evidence that full-fat is better for you than low-fat (even when it doesn't have sugar in it) is compelling.

Dr. Mario Kratz, a nutritional scientist who is based at the Fred Hutchinson Cancer Research Center in Seattle, has looked at an awful lot of studies comparing the benefits of low-fat versus high-fat (i.e., normal, unadulterated) dairy and concluded that "none of the research suggests the low-fat dairy is better." In fact, there are plenty of studies that have found that eating full-fat dairy, particularly yogurt, is likely to lead to less obesity and a lower risk of diseases such as type 2 diabetes.

Yogurt first acquired its healthy aura thanks to Ilya Metchnikoff, a professor at the Pasteur Institute in Paris, who wondered why Bulgarians from the Rhodope Mountains live so much longer than most other Europeans. He decided it was because of bacteria in the yogurt. Dr. Kellogg, who helped found the famous cereal company, was so impressed by this research that he began recommending it to his patients. Except that he suggested they take it as an enema since he thought that was the best way to get it to the large bowel where it would do the most good.

I'm not sure about yogurt enemas, but taken the normal way, through the mouth, there's certainly good evidence that yogurt, with live or active cultures, can help treat conditions like antibiotic-associated diarrhea and IBS, and help reduce constipation. If you want to find out which particular brands have been tested, go to our website.

Another good thing about yogurt is that the fermenting process breaks down lactose so it contains much less than milk. Even if you are lactose-intolerant you should be able to eat yogurt. In fact, eating it can alleviate symptoms.

Cheese

I love cheese but I gave it up for many years because it contains lots of saturated fat and this, I assumed, was likely to lead to an early grave. (I tried eating low-fat cheeses but they tasted terrible.) Then I looked into the science and realized there is no evidence that eating low-fat cheese has any particular health benefits over eating the full-fat version. So I returned to eating proper cheese and have enjoyed every mouthful ever since.

As anyone who has been to France knows, the French eat huge amounts, about 44 pounds per person per year—more than any other country. Yet they have relatively low rates of heart disease and obesity. This is known as the "French paradox." It could be something to do with the fact that they drink lots of wine or maybe there is something special about their lifestyle, but gut bacteria may also play a part.

In a recent study, scientists recruited fifteen healthy young men and asked them to eat lots of cheese and drink full-fat milk on a controlled diet for two weeks. During the weeks when the young men drank milk or ate cheese, there were higher levels of butyrate and propionate in their stools. Both are compounds produced by the biome that have been shown to be good for the gut.[31]

Not all cheese contains live bacteria, and processed cheese contains virtually none. It is important to look for live and active cultures on the food labels. You will find significant numbers of "good" bacteria in Gouda, mozzarella, Cheddar, and cottage cheese, as well as in blue cheese such as Roquefort, though you will need to read the labels to be sure.

One of my other favorite cheeses is feta. It is often made with sheep's or goat milk, and has a lovely creamy, tangy flavor. Feta is rich in a type of bacteria called *Lactobacillus plantarum*, which produces anti-inflammatory compounds. Because it is a fresh cheese made from whole milk it also contains quite a lot of lactose. If you are lactose-intolerant, this may be one to skip.

I love feta in Greek salad (see page 221). It is also delicious grilled or in an omelet with spinach and tomatoes.

Fermented foods

Sauerkraut, kefir, and kimchi

Wine, cheese, yogurt, and chocolate are all fermented foods. That simply means they've been created by microbes converting sugars, such as glucose, into other compounds. The unique flavors and textures you get with different fermented foods are due to the different species of bacteria and yeast involved. I've noticed that sourdough bread made in San Francisco has a completely different taste from sourdough bread made in London and that has to be because the microbes in London are very different from those in San Francisco.

Fermentation has become increasingly popular because it not only adds flavor and texture, but also adds lots of "good" bacteria to your diet. Manufacturers have, of course, jumped on the bandwagon and started selling all sorts of fermented foods. The problem is that many of them have been pasteurized, so there's nothing living in them. I was recently involved in a study in which we sent off a number of store-bought fermented foods, such as sauerkraut and kimchi, to a university to be tested. Sixty percent of the samples we sent grew nothing. You need to buy the products fresh and preferably with some guarantee on the label that they really do contain living bacteria. Or, of course, you could make them yourself.

I'm not familiar with the whole fermenting scene, so I met up with a group of people who are. They're based near London and call themselves The Fermentarium. They are on a mission to spread the word about the joys of making your own fermented food.

When I met Gaba, who is originally from Poland, she was busy making sauerkraut. This is traditionally made from finely shredded cabbage covered in salty water and left to ferment. It is popular in Europe, where it is eaten with sausages or as a side dish.

Gaba learned how to make it from her mother. "My mom, eighty-two, still makes sauerkraut," she told me. "When we were children, living in Poland, she would make a huge vat of sauerkraut in November and put it outside on the balcony where it was well below freezing. When it came to mealtimes she would take a bowl, crack the ice, scoop up some sauerkraut, carry it inside and warm it up. And that vat of sauerkraut would see us through until the spring."

Gaba said that while most people, particularly at first, tend to stick to fermenting milk or vegetables, you can ferment almost anything, including pork fat and raw fish.

At this point I had a flashback of one of the most revolting foods I have ever eaten, and that was fermented shark. I was in Iceland and because it is something of a tradition there I thought I would give it a go. Big mistake. I got one mouthful down before I started to gag. This is strictly for hard-core fermenters, though at least the fermented shark they eat these days is produced more hygienically than it used to be. In the good old days, I was told, you would take your freshly caught shark, put it in a bucket, urinate over it, add some salty water, and then leave it somewhere in the basement to ferment until it was time for the party to begin. Which could be months.

Gaba assured me she never goes that far when she is fermenting fish. "We don't do it to the point that the Icelanders and Norwegians do, not until it is rotten. We just ferment for a couple of days."

Gaba adores the smells and flavors that you get only from fermented food. She wondered why fermented foods aren't a larger part of our culture. "You make cider, apple cider vinegar, bread, and cheese, but as a nation you seem to be very reluctant to eat, let alone make, the more exotic and vinegary rich foods that are found widely in Eastern Europe and farther east."

She thinks one of the main reasons why Eastern Europeans are keen on fermented food is that they have to endure much longer and colder winters. In earlier times it was almost impossible to buy vegetables for much of the year. That's why peasants, before the days of refrigeration, found so many different ways to pickle and preserve food.

The homemade sauerkraut Gaba had brought along for me to taste was delicious and nothing like the vinegary stuff from supermarkets that I'd tried before. Freshly made sauerkraut is packed full of live bacteria and surprisingly easy to make. There's a recipe for sauerkraut on page 257, as well as one for kefir (a fermented milk drink, which offers one of the most probiotic-rich concoctions available) on page 208.

Kimchi, a spicy Korean side dish made from vegetables, is another popular fermented food. I read somewhere that kimchi is going to be this year's Hot Ingredient, being added to everything from tacos to pizza, even to a grilled-cheese sandwich. It's versatile and packs a punch. Are your taste buds and microbiome ready for it? Try it and see.

One of the reasons fermented foods are so good for the gut is that, ounce for ounce, they contain a huge number of different microbes. The microbes in fermented foods are also far more likely than most other bacteria to make it safely down into your colon because they are extremely resistant to acid, having been reared in an acidic environment. You might worry about the impact on your gut of eating foods which are acidic, like sauerkraut and kimchi, but all the evidence shows that they are good for you. Do, however, start slowly if you haven't eaten these sorts of foods before.

Apple cider vinegar

You may not have come across kimchi or kefir, but you probably have tried apple cider vinegar. This is another fermented food that is now hugely popular, and we have included a number of recipes that contain it.

The actress Scarlett Johansson apparently washes her face with a diluted version of the stuff, while the Arctic explorer Sir Ranulph Fiennes also swears by it, claiming he beat his arthritis thanks to a vinegary drink (four parts apple cider vinegar to one part raw honey).

More heavyweight endorsement comes from Hippocrates of Kos, often described as the "Father of Modern Medicine." Hippocrates was a great believer in the power of the body to heal itself. To help the body on its way he often prescribed vinegar and fasting. He described fasting as the "physician within" and claimed that "to eat when you are sick is to feed your sickness." As for vinegar, he recommended its use for a wide range of things, from cleaning wounds to sorting out a persistent cough. But does it really have any remarkable health-giving properties?

I recently teamed up with Dr. James Brown from Aston University in Birmingham, England, to find out. The first thing we decided to test was the claim that drinking a couple of tablespoons of vinegar before a meal will help control your blood sugar levels and prevent blood sugar spikes.

We started by recruiting some healthy volunteers and asked them to eat a bagel. James measured their blood sugar levels before and after.

As expected, bagel consumption was followed by a large and rapid rise in their blood sugar levels. The next day we asked them to eat another bagel, but this time they had to knock back a shot of diluted apple cider vinegar just before doing so. This reduced the amount of sugar going into our volunteers' blood by almost 50 percent.

James was delighted with this finding. "There have been studies which suggest this happens in people who are at high risk of diabetes," he told me, "but I'm not sure it's been shown in healthy volunteers before so I was pleasantly surprised."

This probably happens because the acetic acid in the vinegar suppresses the activity of an enzyme called disaccharidase, which breaks down starches and complex sugars, enabling them to be more rapidly absorbed by the body. If the enzyme is blocked, far less sugar gets absorbed.

But would apple cider vinegar drinkers come out better in other measures, such as weight loss, lower cholesterol, or reduced inflammation?

James divided volunteers into three groups. For eight weeks, the first group had to consume two tablespoons of apple cider vinegar just before lunch and dinner, either mixed with water or on a salad. The second group was asked to do the same with malt vinegar and the final group got vinegary-smelling water (placebo).

By the end of eight weeks none of them had lost any weight, though the apple cider drinkers were very positive about the experience. A woman with mild arthritis told me, "I have had less aches and pains in my joints, especially after exercise."

As part of the testing James had measured their levels of CRP, the marker for inflammation in the body. He didn't find major changes across the groups, although some of the apple cider vinegar drinkers did have falls in their CRP levels. What he did see, which surprised him, was quite a big change in cholesterol, but only in the apple cider vinegar drinkers.

In this group there was an average 10 percent reduction in total cholesterol, with a particularly big reduction in triglycerides (a form of fat carried in the blood). This was a striking finding because our volunteers were all healthy at the start, with normal cholesterol levels.

The fact that we only saw this effect with the apple cider

vinegar, and not with the group drinking malt vinegar, suggests that the apples are playing a special role.

"Apple cider vinegar has lots of different, bioactive molecules which are found in apples," James said, "and at least two of those molecules have been shown to have really beneficial effects. So it's likely that there is a component in apples found in a concentrated form in apple cider vinegar which has given us this result."

In this particular experiment we didn't look at the participants' stool, but other studies have suggested that apple cider vinegar can be good for the stomach as well as blood sugar and cholesterol levels. That said, it is not a cure-all and it is really acidic, so I wouldn't recommend splashing it on your face or glugging it down neat. Drink it diluted or use it sparingly in your food. I personally like it on salad, as a vinaigrette.

Clever Gut Apple Cider Vinaigrette

1 tablespoon French mustard
1 garlic clove, crushed
2 tablespoons apple cider vinegar
1 tablespoon balsamic vinegar
6 tablespoons olive oil

Other uses for apple cider vinegar that I've heard of but not personally tested include:

- Wart removal—soak a cotton pad with vinegar and secure it over the wart. Leave it on overnight, and repeat every day for a week.

- Curing bad breath—add 1½ teaspoons to a cup of water, and gargle.

- Soothing a sore throat—mix 2 tablespoons with 2 tablespoons warm water and gargle.

- Shiny hair—add 4 tablespoons to a cup of water and pour it over your hair after shampooing. Leave it on for a moment and then rinse.

Probiotic supplements

As well as getting them in fresh foods, you can get probiotics in the form of capsules, pills, or processed foods that contain live bacteria. There is a huge market for probiotics, many of which are overhyped, like fish oil capsules. The response of most of the experts I've spoken to has been skepticism, particularly when it comes to so-called probiotic yogurts. These are yogurts with "added bacteria." The clever thing the manufacturers did was fund research into the potential health benefits of their products, on the back of which they were heavily promoted around the world.

But when scientists from the European Food Safety Authority looked at some of these claims (for UK yogurt brands Yakult and Actimel) they were not convinced. On their websites, you will see they mention that their products contain lots of *Lactobacillus*, but they are careful not to make specific health claims.

I personally avoid all such products, not least because they tend to contain extra sugar or sweeteners. But if I had a particular condition I wanted treated, such as antibiotic-induced diarrhea, I might take a proper probiotic.

Graeme Close, professor of human physiology at Liverpool John Moores University, certainly thinks that probiotics, targeted at specific problems, are worth considering. As well as doing his university work, he advises the England rugby team, Everton Football Club, and the European Tour golfers on what to eat. He says that when his teams are all together in camp, training hard, taking a good probiotic may reduce the risk of them coming down with something nasty.

"What we find," he said, "in elite athletes is that, after an intense exercise session, you can experience temporary damage to the gut, which creates a window of opportunity for pathogens, 'bad' bacteria, to take hold. If you are training hard, day after day, you get these spikes of increased vulnerability."

This could explain why elite athletes are often ill before a big event. When world champion runner Paula Radcliffe went for Olympic gold in Athens, she was thwarted by a bout of severe diarrhea during the race.

To minimize the risk of this happening, Graeme recommends taking a multi-strain probiotic if you are doing heavy training (for more details, go to our website). Graeme also recommends taking vitamin D supplements, particularly during the winter months, because low levels of vitamin D are bad for the biome.

"I don't recommend many supplements. I believe in food first," Graeme assured me. "In sports nutrition this has changed enormously. If you were in pro sports ten years ago you could have been taking dozens of supplements."

For the scientific evidence behind a wide range of probiotic supplements, I recommend you go to Medline Plus, a service provided by the American National Library of Medicine, which brings together reliable information from the National Institutes of Health as well as other health-related organizations: medlineplus.gov/druginfo/natural /790.html. (And see page 270.)

Foods to avoid

As well as things you should eat, there are also things you should cut down on and preferably avoid if you want a healthy, diverse biome. Top of my list are sugar and processed food.

Sugar

The high-sugar diet that many of us have been indulging in has had a catastrophic effect on our health. In the UK the average six-year-old eats his or her own weight in sugar every year, and attempts to curb this have been largely unsuccessful. If you still think that sugar is a bit of harmless fun then let me spoil your day by listing some of the downsides of this pure, white, and deadly substance:

1. Sugar contains no essential ingredients. None. It's just calories. Other foods may have traces of vitamins, minerals, fiber . . . something. Sugar does not.

2. Sugar rots your teeth. I've had almost every tooth in my face filled and drilled because when I was a child I ate and drank too much sugar. One reason children under ten are admitted to the hospital is to have their severely rotten teeth extracted.

3. Eating or drinking sugar causes your blood sugar levels to spike, then crash, which makes you hungry. People who eat a lot of sugary things tend to be fatter. This is particularly true of children. One study found that drinking a single sugar-sweetened drink per day increased the risk of becoming obese by around 60 percent.[32]

4. Because of its effect on your weight and on your insulin levels, consuming lots of sugar puts you at increased risk of type 2 diabetes. This can lead to dementia and amputation. Being a diabetic also cuts ten years off your life, despite medication.

5. Sugar is addictive. Not, oddly enough, on its own. I don't dive into the sugar bowl. It's when sugar is mixed with fat, in that ratio of one calorie of sugar to one calorie of fat, that we find it irresistible. There are some people who can take a sliver of cake and leave the rest, but there are plenty more who can't.

Food and drink manufacturers, who have spent years funding research to show that sugar is absolutely fine (a tactic reminiscent of the tobacco industry), are well aware that the tide is turning. So they have begun vigorous attempts to sell us low- or zero-calorie alternatives. But are these alternatives any healthier? The jury is out, but evidence is mounting that they are not.

The whole point of zero-calorie sweeteners is that they give you the taste of sugar without the calories. But your body and brain are not so easily fooled. A study on fruit flies, done by researchers from the University of Sydney, showed how artificial sweeteners lead to changes in parts of the brain which regulate appetite.[33]

They found that fruit flies consumed 30 percent more calories after eating artificial sweeteners than after a food sweetened with normal sugar. So what's going on?

Researcher Greg Neely explained, "When sweetness versus energy is out of balance for a period of time, the brain recalibrates and increases total calories consumed."

In other words, if your brain thinks you are about to get a sugar hit (because your taste buds tell it that sugar is on the way), but nothing arrives, then it will eventually decide you need to eat something else to compensate.

Fruit flies, of course, are not human, but these findings are in line with other studies that have shown that consuming artificial sweeteners, mainly in the form of carbonated drinks, is no better for you, and may even be worse, than taking your sugar straight.

That was certainly the conclusion of a big meta-analysis, looking at a whole range of recent studies.[34]

Artificial sweeteners

As well as affecting your brain, artificial sweeteners can change your gut bacteria.

A few years ago the two Erans from the Weizmann Institute, whom we met earlier, Dr. Eran Elinav and Dr. Eran Segal, did experiments looking at the impact of consuming artificial sweeteners on the biome.[35]

Mice were given water, sugary water, or water laced with saccharin to drink. Unlike those that drank water or sugary water, the mice that got the saccharin soon developed glucose intolerance, a step on the way to diabetes.

Next, they transferred the biome from the mice that had consumed saccharin to "germ-free," or sterile, mice. Within six days these mice had also developed glucose intolerance, suggesting that there was something in the transplanted biome that had been changed by the sweetener. A closer look at their stool confirmed that their guts now had more of the sort of bacteria that lead to obesity and diabetes and less of our Old Friend, *Akkermansia*.

Finally, they asked a group of human volunteers, who normally didn't eat or drink artificially sweetened foods, to consume a high, but safe, dose for a week.

Within seven days many, but not all, of the volunteers began to develop signs of glucose intolerance. Why? Well it appears that some gut bacteria react to sweeteners by secreting chemicals that provoke an inflammatory response, which in turn encourages obesity and diabetes. If you have those sorts of bacteria, sweeteners should definitely be off the menu. How can you find out if you have them? At the moment you can't. I steer clear of artificial sweeteners and would recommend you do as well.

Dr. Elinav, who is clearly not a fan of artificial sweeteners, thinks that there should be a "reassessment of today's massive, unsupervised consumption of these substances."

So what's the alternative?

Unfortunately, natural alternatives to sugar, like honey and agave syrup, will have a similar effect on your blood sugar levels as eating sugar. I'm not totally against them, but they are a wolf in sheep's clothing.

The trouble is, I still like the sweet stuff. So I was intrigued when someone suggested I try the extract of an African fruit, *Synsepalum dulcificum,* better known as the miracle berry. Miracle berries contain miraculin, a molecule that binds to receptors on your tongue, changing their shape. Miracle berries are unlike any other sweetener because they work not by making foods sweeter but by making them *taste* sweeter.

Fresh berries are hard to get your hands on, but you can buy the dehydrated pulp of the fresh berries in tablet form on the internet.

So what are they like? I put one on my tongue, waited for it to dissolve, and then I was good to go. I had read enthusiastic claims that it made foods, such as oranges, taste as if they had been "freshly plucked from the Garden of Eden."

The tablet I tried certainly took the bitter edge off licking a lemon, but the aftertaste was unpleasant. An expensive red wine was transformed by it into something that was disgustingly sweet and fizzy. The only good thing was that the effects wore off within an hour.

Grasping the nettle

If you have a sweet tooth and are worried that you are downing too much sugary stuff, I suspect "cold turkey" is the way to go. But rather than rely on will power it's important to find something else to fill the void.

The Australian actress Rebel Wilson managed to lose about 33 pounds by ditching sugary snacks and increasing the amount of fiber she ate. She also started doing five to ten minutes of high intensity training (HIT) four times a week.

According to reliable sources (i.e., a celebrity website), Rebel aims for 35 grams (about 1¼ ounces) of fiber a day, which she gets by eating oatmeal, fruits, veggies, and whole grains. When she feels a craving for sugar she has a shot of organic apple cider vinegar.

Rather than eating pretzels, bagels, and bread, she now fills up on healthy fats such as olive oil and avocado. Her go-to snacks include:

Carrot and cucumber sticks dipped in guacamole
Almond butter on celery and carrots
A handful of almonds, Brazil nuts, or cashews

Like Rebel, I snack on nuts and veggies when the desire for cake or chocolate becomes almost unbearable. I also find it useful to imagine that I am slowly starving out those sugar-hungry microbes in my gut. Man versus microbe. Surely there can only be one winner? If you want more advice about how and why you should cut down on sugar visit thebloodsugardiet.com.

155

Processed foods

A couple of years ago Tim Spector, professor of genetic epidemiology at King's College, London, persuaded his son Tom to go on a fast-food diet. For ten days Tom ate nothing but the food he could buy from his local McDonald's. This included lots of Big Macs, chicken nuggets, and fries, all washed down with Coke. Before, during, and after, samples of Tom's stool were sent off to be analyzed. Understandably, Tom did not feel great on this diet, and his gut biome had an even worse time. After a few days he had lost around 1,400 species, roughly 40 percent of his total. Weeks after returning to his normal diet his biome still hadn't recovered.[36]

A few years ago I did a similar, albeit less extreme self-experiment. To see how bad a diet of processed food could be, I decided to go on one for four weeks—not living entirely on McDonald's like Tom, just eating processed meat once or twice a day.

On this new regimen, I started most mornings with a couple of bits of bacon. I then had a salad for lunch and a small burger for my evening meal. On another day, perhaps a sausage for breakfast and a salami sandwich for lunch. In many ways it was a fairly typical British diet.

To monitor the impact of this, before I started I went to the Food and Nutritional Sciences Department at Reading University. They gave me a thorough health check, measuring my cholesterol, weight, body fat, and blood pressure and taking stool samples.

Four weeks later I returned.

When I stepped on the scales the nurse, with a slight smile, said I had put on an impressive 6½ pounds since my last visit, much of it around my gut. This was bad news because fat around your abdomen greatly increases your risk of becoming insulin-resistant and diabetic.

Then I had my blood pressure taken. Yet more bad news. I had gone from "excellent" to "stage 1 hypertensive."

My gut bacteria had also changed, in a bad direction.

My diversity score (which is one of the better measures of general gut health) had fallen from 7.27 to 7.1 (where 10 is the most diverse). This doesn't sound like much but it meant that whereas previously I had had a reassuringly diverse microbiome (I was in the top 30 percent), now I had fallen right down the rankings and was languishing in the bottom 30 percent.

There was also a major shift in my gut bacteria in favor of *Firmicutes*, the sort of bacteria that are linked to obesity and inflammation. After reverting to my normal diet my weight, blood pressure, and biome gradually returned to normal.

It's not surprising that processed food is bad for you, but it is striking just how bad it is for your biome. One reason is the amount of sugar and fat in processed food, but there is also the matter of emulsifiers.

Emulsifiers, which are a sort of detergent, are added to most processed foods for texture and to extend their shelf life. Feeding common emulsifiers to mice tilts their biome in an unhealthy direction and encourages the growth of bacteria that attack the mucous lining of the gut. This in turn leads to inflammation, which contributes to the development of diseases like type 2 diabetes and obesity.[37]

Another good reason to say no to burgers and fries.

Antibiotics

When I was a child we lived in India. While we were there I had multiple bouts of severe diarrhea, which in turn meant numerous courses of antibiotics. These almost certainly saved my life, but may have contributed to the fact that I later developed type 2 diabetes (which I then overcame, see Chapter 6).

Many children are exposed to antibiotics before they are born. Pregnant women are routinely prescribed them, and they readily cross the placenta and reach the fetus. The mother of a baby who is going to be born by Cesarean section will also routinely get antibiotics, which will do nothing good for that baby's biome. The baby will already have a greater risk of developing asthma and type 1 diabetes than one born vaginally, as we saw in Chapter 4, and this early exposure to antibiotics may increase that risk.

The first two to three years of life are hugely important, not just for a growing child but also for their microbiome. That's when it gets established. Repeated doses of broad-spectrum antibiotics like penicillin, given in those first few years, significantly increase the risk of developing type 2 diabetes and becoming obese.

Some experts recommend that if a young child has to have antibiotics, then it would be a good idea to take a course of probiotics at the same time, possibly with some fermented food like yogurt or kefir as well. The same is true if you have to take a course of antibiotics as an adult. It's advice that Sophie Ramsbotham wishes someone had given her.

Sophie's story

Sophie is twenty-nine years old and works as a garden designer. When she was in her early twenties she lived in India, designing classrooms for special-needs children. While she was there she got typhoid fever.

A prolonged course of antibiotics dealt with the immediate problem and she returned home to the US. But over the next two years she struggled with terrible gut problems. These included pain, bloating, and frequent diarrhea. She was often bedridden and had to drop out of college where she was studying architecture. She saw a lot of doctors.

"At least twenty, and to be honest none of them had a clue of what to do," she told me. "They clearly felt pretty hopeless. They kept suggesting more tests, more invasive endoscopic procedures, more antibiotics. I was also told, 'You have IBS, go and deal with it.'"

She ended up, reluctantly, visiting a neurologist, who also described himself as a "functional doctor." He offered to heal her through diet.

"There were lots more blood tests. Lots of stool tests. He found plenty of nasties in my gut which he tried to kill with monolaurin (a substance derived from coconut that has antimicrobial properties)."

He also put her on a radical diet. His approach was to take out all the foods that might be a problem.

"I was down to chicken, sweet potatoes, and broccoli. That was it. I was also taking lots of supplements to try and heal up the lining of my gut."

The good news was that, for the first time in many years, her guts felt better. The bad news was, on her incredibly restrictive diet, she still felt run-down, tired, and lethargic most of the time.

She moved, with her husband, to London where she found Tanya Borowski.

"Under Tanya's guidance I started to expand my diet again, eat things like lentils and grains. I don't think I will ever be back on dairy. These days we eat a lot of sauerkraut and kombucha which we make ourselves. My husband wants to get into kimchi. If I had to take antibiotics again I would also take high doses of probiotics and eat lots of fermented foods as well. No one tells you that. I wish they had."

We love homemade yogurt because it usually has a higher probiotic content than store-bought versions—it's much tastier, too.

Homemade Yogurt, page 206

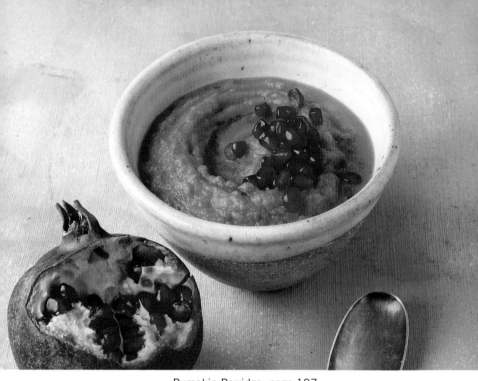

Pumpkin Porridge, page 197;
Breakfast Bread with Raspberry Chia Jam, page 211; Chia Pot, page 201

Classic Greek Salad, page 221; Green Pea Soup, page 221;
Walnut and Red Pepper Dip, page 214; Chocolate Eggplant Brownies, page 259

Phytonutrients are the natural components of plants that keep them healthy. Their antioxidant and anti-inflammatory properties help to preserve the microbial balance in the gut, keeping it in good working order.

Phyto Burst Lunch Box, page 226

The magic ingredients of Tanya's
Gut-soothing Bone Broth, page 216

Chicken Goujons with Hummus, page 244; Asian Coleslaw with Chicken, page 235;
Harissa and Beet Salmon, page 245; Cod in Salsa Verde, page 246

Baked Rainbow Ratatoullie, page 254

Foods to enjoy on the
Clever Gut Diet

Other Ways to Improve Your Biome

Intermittent fasting

Back in 2012 I discovered, through a random blood test, that I was a type 2 diabetic. Rather than start on medication I decided to see if there was any way to reverse this. I spoke to lots of scientists and came across something I'd never heard about before, intermittent fasting.

Intermittent fasting doesn't mean cutting out food altogether. It means reducing your calories, fairly dramatically, a couple of days a week. Intrigued, I made a documentary called *Eat, Fast, Live Longer*, with myself as a guinea pig. As part of the documentary I decided to see what would happen if I cut my calorie intake to around 600 a day for two days a week, and did this for eight weeks.

I found it surprisingly easy to do, and on what I was now calling a 5:2 diet I lost 22 pounds, reversed my diabetes, and took four inches off my waist. Based on my experience, and numerous conversations with experts, I wrote *The FastDiet*, which became an international bestseller. This turned intermittent fasting into a worldwide phenomenon, and garnered fans including Jennifer Lopez and Benedict Cumberbatch. Five years on, I've maintained both the weight loss and the improved blood sugar levels.

So why does it work?

One reason why the 5:2 has been so successful is that you aren't on a constant treadmill, dieting all the time. It's easier to resist the temptation to eat something unhealthy if you say to yourself, "I will have it tomorrow." Then tomorrow comes and maybe you eat it. But often you don't.

Intermittent fasting also teaches you better ways of eating. If you satisfy your hunger on fasting days by eating vegetables and good protein, then over time you'll discover that when you get hungry you are more likely to crave the healthy stuff.

The science behind it is strong and getting stronger. A recent review article published in the scientific journal *Cell Metabolism*, "Fasting: Molecular Mechanisms and Clinical Applications," looked at numerous human and animal studies and concluded that intermittent fasting reduces many of the things that encourage aging (oxidative damage and inflammation) while increasing the body's ability to protect and repair itself. According to this article it "helps reduce obesity, hypertension, asthma, and rheumatoid arthritis."

Fasting and the gut

If it is doing good things to your body, what effect is it having on your microbiome? Well, there is one species of bacteria we've met before that flourishes when we cut our calories or don't eat anything: *Akkermansia*.

Because *Akkermansia* lives on mucus and not on the remains of the food you've eaten, as most gut microbes do, it thrives when you reduce your calories. In the cutthroat world of the gut, *Akkermansia* has the upper hand in situations where its rivals are short of nourishment.

As well as animal studies, there have been a couple of small-scale human studies that have shown this. In one,[38] thirteen overweight men and women were asked to go on a low-calorie diet for a week, eating 600 to 800 calories a day.

Stool samples were taken at the beginning and end of the week. The main finding was an increase in microbial diversity (which, as we've seen, is a good thing), and a dramatic rise in *Akkermansia* and *Bifidobacterium* (also good guys).

In another small study[39] researchers from the American Gut project put nineteen volunteers through a cheese and yogurt diet, a dietary cleanse (fruit and vegetable smoothies or water with lemon, maple syrup, and cayenne pepper), or fasting (water only or minimal calories). They took stool samples every day for the three days of the study and for a week afterward.

Going on a fast was the most effective way to change the biome. It led to big increases in *Akkermansia*, which persisted for about ten days after the fast had ended. Levels then slowly dropped back to where they had started.

So a short fasting blast can kick-start changes, but if you want to maintain those changes you may need to keep doing a bit of calorie restriction once a week or so (I call it 6:1, and that's what I do).

As well as being a professor of epidemiology, Dr. Tim Spector, whom we met earlier, is a founder of the British Gut project and a leading microbiome researcher. Like me, he is a huge fan of the Mediterranean diet. "It is the only one that has been proven to be beneficial for health," he says. "Nuts, seeds, dark chocolate, red wine, olive oil, and vegetables like leeks, garlic, and onions are packed with the chemicals that microbes love. We should also be eating more fermented foods like live yogurt, kimchi, sauerkraut, and kefir."

Furthermore, he thinks that highly restrictive diets, which cut out whole food groups, such as Atkins, are likely to be bad for the biome. In fact, the only "diet" he agrees with is intermittent fasting, preferably with a high fiber intake. "I like your 5:2 plan," he told me, "because it keeps food intake diverse."

People often misinterpret the 5:2 approach, claiming that it allows you to eat "whatever you like" on the days that you are not fasting. This is not true. The best way to do 5:2 is to go on a Mediterranean-style diet, reducing your calories two days a week. I'm not rigid about the number of calories for the fasting days. Some people find they get by comfortably on 600 calories. Others struggle. If you find that 600 calories leave you starving, then increase to 800 calories.

For more information on the science and how to do it, read *The FastDiet* or visit thefastdiet.co.uk or thebloodsugardiet.com, where you will find a vibrant and supportive community of happy fasters.

Exercise

We know that exercise and increased activity are essential to keep your heart in good shape and your brain ticking over. More surprisingly, exercise also seems to be good for your biome.

Evidence for this comes from a study done by the Microbiome Institute in Cork, Ireland, where researchers decided to take a close look at the stool of the Irish rugby team.

Dr. Paul Cotter, one of the researchers, told me the reason they did the study with the rugby team was that they were an exceptional group of athletes. "We thought that if this particular group of young men didn't have an altered gut microbiota then no one's gut microbiota would be altered by exercise." So what did they find?

"The rugby guys had a weird microbiota, hugely diverse," Paul said. "We have only seen comparable results from people living in the Amazon rain forest or hunter-gatherers like the Hadza."

This study provided the first real evidence that exercise increases microbial diversity in humans. Paul decided to follow it up by looking at the impact of exercise on people who don't usually do a lot of exercise.

"What we did," Paul told me, "was take a group of couch potatoes, and put them through an eight-week exercise regimen. While they were doing the training we also gave them whey protein, because adding protein seems to be important. We took samples before, during, and after, looking primarily for changes in their gut diversity."

The study isn't yet fully complete, let alone published, but Paul is quietly excited. "We didn't think we would see much in that short a time period; we thought it would merely be a stepping stone for a bigger study, but I've started crunching the data and we are already seeing some intriguing changes."

Paul thinks that exercise will almost certainly help make your biome healthier but he also told me, "You can't outrun a bad diet."

As well as doing lots of exercise the Irish rugby players were eating a rich and varied diet. After training they would go to a special buffet where they ate lots of fruits, vegetables, white meat, nuts, berries, seeds, that sort of thing. The days of a beer and a pie after training are over for elite athletes.

So if you want to improve your biome, what type of exercise and how long? The honest answer is that we don't know but it is likely that anything will help; running, walking, swimming, taking the stairs, even just standing around more will probably make a difference. Above all, avoid sitting around too much.

As someone who makes documentaries for a living, I regret having to tell you this, but television kills. Professor David Spiegelhalter of Cambridge University has calculated that every two hours you spend sitting down watching TV cuts your life expectancy by about half an hour. The other problem is that if you are sitting down watching TV you are also probably eating potato chips and other junk food.

One way around this is to watch TV standing up (perhaps doing the ironing, which burns about 80 calories an hour) or while on an exercise bike.

For optimal health you also need to inject some intensity into your exercise. The type of exercise I favor is high intensity training (HIT). For me this means very short bursts on a bike or just running up a flight of stairs, anywhere I can really push myself.

This seems to be a particularly efficient way of building up the strength of your heart and lungs—even if you manage just a few minutes a week.

So how does HIT work? One of the things it does more effectively than low intensity exercise is stimulate your mitochondria—the body's main power plants. Their job is to convert raw materials such as oxygen and glucose into little packages of energy called adenosine triphosphate (ATP). The ATP is then used to power your body.

There are mitochondria in every cell of your body and, since they produce power, you want more of them. A good measure of how effective an exercise regimen is going to be is whether it results in greater mitochondrial density.

That's where HIT scores particularly well. Doing HIT leads to greater numbers of more active mitochondria than standard exercise, and this is particularly impressive when it comes to heart muscle. HIT makes the heart bigger, stronger, and more efficient. This is important not only if you are going for a run, but also if you are recovering from a heart attack.

In addition, mitochondria are crucial to fat-burning. When you start to exercise, your body breaks down the fat stores, releasing free fatty acids into your blood. These fatty acids are taken up by the muscle and converted by the mitochondria into energy. The more mitochondria you have, the greater the fat consumption.

Compared with people on standard exercise regimens, those who do HIT see a bigger loss in abdominal fat, which as well as being unsightly is a risk factor for diabetes and heart disease.

A few years ago I wrote a book called *FastExercise*, which extolled the virtues of HIT. Although people were enthusiastic about the science, there was also anxiety about the risks associated with pushing yourself hard, particularly if you are a bit older.

So I am delighted by a recent study, "Extremely short-duration high-intensity training substantially improves the physical function and self-reported health status of an elderly population," published in the *Journal of the American Geriatrics Society*.[40]

In this study, scientists from Abertay University in Scotland put a group of unfit, elderly volunteers through an exercise regimen in which they were expected to do two minutes of HIT a week. The volunteers ranged in age from sixty-one to seventy-four.

The volunteers, untrained individuals who had done no regular exercise over the previous year, were screened to make sure they weren't on any medication that would affect their performance. Then they were randomly allocated into an exercise or control group.

The two sessions consisted of 10 x 6 seconds of all-out sprints against resistance on an exercise bike, with at least one minute to recover between each sprint. They wore a heart monitor and were asked not to do another sprint until their heart rate had dropped back to below 120 beats per second.

The secret to doing HIT is not speed, but effort. You have to push yourself, which means doing it on something like an exercise bike, where you quickly increase resistance. As Dr. John Babraj, the lead scientist put it, "When it comes to the sprints, you don't have to go at the speed of someone like Usain Bolt. As long as you are putting in your maximal effort—whatever speed that happens to be—it will improve your health."

By the end of the six-week trial, the volunteers doing their two minutes of HIT a week had lost an average of 2 pounds, mostly fat, despite having been asked not to change their eating habits. Dr. Babraj thinks this is partly due to an afterburn effect you get from doing HIT, an increase in metabolic rate that persists for many hours. It is not much, around 70 calories a day, but over six weeks that would add up to around 2,000 calories, the energy equivalent of about 10 ounces of fat. Unlike conventional exercise, which tends to lead to compensatory overeating, HIT also seems to suppress appetite.

The real benefits of his two-minute exercise regimen, for the more mature of us, were seen in its effect on blood pressure, aerobic fitness, and blood glucose. High blood pressure is a significant risk factor for heart disease and stroke.

The volunteers doing HIT had an average drop in blood pressure of around 9 percent, better than you would get with most drugs. They saw a similar drop in their blood glucose.

They also saw an 8 percent improvement in aerobic fitness, which is a measure of the strength of your heart and lungs. Aerobic fitness is one of the most accurate predictors of how well and how long we will live.

Clearly people who are older need to take things more gently when they start, but there is a persistent and overstated fear that exercise in later life will lead to heart attacks and strokes. The reverse is true. However, if you are on medication or are worried about your health do consult your doctor before starting a new exercise regimen.

The dangers of overdoing it

Although not doing any exercise is bad for you, there are dangers in overdoing things, even when you are fit. A lot of runners who really push themselves have gut problems, particularly after doing something strenuous like a marathon. I'm told, though I've never done one, that the biggest queues at these events are for the bathroom. "Marathons are won and lost in the toilet," I was informed by a friend. The problem is that excessive exercise can lead to gut damage and leaky gut syndrome. The damage to the gut is caused by an increase in body temperature and a reduction in blood flow. In most people it seems to be only a temporary effect, but just be aware that though modest levels of exercise will improve your gut, it won't enjoy being pushed too far.

Stress, sleep, and the biome

One of the things that exercise is good for is relieving stress. Too much stress, lack of sleep, and an unhealthy biome are all interlinked.

Stress makes you sleep badly, which makes you eat badly (it cranks up your desire for sugary carbs and high-fat snacks), which encourages the growth of "bad" microbes in your gut. You put on weight, get crankier, sleep even worse, and so on and so on. It is a horrible, vicious cycle. The immediate effects of a bad night's sleep are particularly striking when it comes to appetite.

In one study in which they asked twenty-seven men and women (aged thirty to forty-five) to cut down their sleep to four hours for just one night, they found dramatic changes in their hunger hormones and appetite.[41] Oddly enough, sleep deprivation affected men and women differently. In the case of the men, the reduced sleep led to a surge in the hormone ghrelin, which tells you that you are hungry.

In the women that didn't happen. Instead, there was a fall in a hormone called GLP-1, which tells you when you are full. The effect was the same, the subjects ate more, but for different reasons. It's not clear why there is this gender split.

Shift work and jet lag also do pretty awful things to your body and your biome. On a recent filming trip I got chatting with a flight attendant who told me she survives on sleeping pills and energy drinks. She knows this is a terrible combination, but she's in a rut. "I haven't told my husband," she confided. "He thinks I'm taking iron tablets last thing at night."

The Erans (Dr. Elinav and Dr. Segal), the brains behind the Personalized Nutrition Project, decided to explore this and asked some students to fly across time zones. Naturally enough, they were also asked to collect their own feces samples before they got on the plane, later when their jet lag was particularly bad, and then two weeks after that.

The Erans then transferred the bacteria from the students into germ-free mice. Dr. Elinav says the results were startling. "The mice that received the microbes from jet-lagged students grew obese and developed diabetes. Those that were given bacteria from samples taken before or after the jet lag set in were unaffected."

The moral is, try to avoid flying across lots of time zones, if you can. The other moral is prioritize a good night's sleep. Easier said than done.

If you are sleep deprived, what can you do about it?

There's plenty of sleep advice out there, most of which I've tried and some of which has helped. The best-tested, scientifically based advice includes the following:

1. Set your alarm clock to wake you up at the same time every morning. This creates a ritual and your body loves rituals. Sadly, that means no weekend sleep-ins.

2. Try to go for a walk before breakfast. Morning light switches off your brain's production of melatonin, the hormone that helps put you to sleep. Bright light really will perk you up. If you suffer from seasonal affective disorder (the winter blues) this will be particularly helpful.

3. Do some exercise during the day. Lots of studies show that exercise improves quality of sleep.

4. Prepare for sleep at least ninety minutes before you go to bed. Eating late at night is really bad for your body and forcing your gut to do lots of heavy digestive work is not going to improve the quality of your sleep.

5. Having a warm bath or hot shower at least an hour before going to bed can also be helpful, as long as you cool down afterward. It is the drop in body temperature that cues your brain that it is time to sleep. That is also why you should try to sleep in a cool room.

6. Avoid watching TV, being on your phone or social media in the run-up to bedtime. This is partly because these activities are overly stimulating, but also because the blue light screens typically emit will wake your brain up. Do not, whatever you do, watch TV or use your laptop in bed. Bed should be for sleeping and sex, nothing else.

7. Cut down on late-night boozing. Alcohol may help you go to sleep but it will also ruin your REM sleep. Whether or not you choose to drink coffee in the evening is a more individual thing. Some people are fast caffeine metabolizers, meaning they have a gene that breaks down caffeine particularly fast. I've been tested; I'm a fast metabolizer and drinking coffee at night makes very little difference to my sleep quality. My wife, on the other hand, is a slow metabolizer and can't drink coffee after lunch or she will sleep really badly.

8. Before you go to sleep, write down three good things that happened to you that day. This has been shown to be one of the best ways to improve mood.

That's the well-established stuff, which if you are an insomniac you have probably already tried. You may also have tried lavender or other herbal remedies. The evidence for these is weak, but they may work for you.

Now let's move on to one of the more surprising approaches to improving your sleep patterns: changing your biome.

Fiber and sleep

Eating fiber, as we've seen, increases levels of "good" bacteria, such as *Bifidobacteria*, which in turn produce all sorts of hormones and metabolites that improve not only your gut health, and your weight but also, possibly, your brain. There is now evidence that more fiber will help you sleep better, too.

In a recent study researchers from the Institute of Human Nutrition at Columbia University Medical Center in New York brought thirteen men and thirteen women, average age thirty-five, into their sleep clinic and tested different diets on them. These included changing the amounts of fiber, saturated fat, and sugar in the meals they were eating.[42]

What they found was that having meals rich in fiber improved the quality of the volunteers' deep sleep and also meant they got to sleep faster (down from an average of twenty-nine minutes to seventeen minutes). Eating more saturated fat and sugar, on the other hand, led to poorer-quality sleep—it was lighter and less refreshing.

As Dr. Marie-Pierre St-Onge, one of the main researchers, pointed out, "The finding that diet can influence sleep has tremendous health implications, given the increasing recognition of the role of sleep in the development of chronic disorders such as hypertension, diabetes, and cardiovascular disease."

Potato starch and sleep

As well as cramming in more vegetables, I've been trying a type of fiber that *Bifidobacteria* seem to particularly like—potato starch. Potato starch is a form of resistant starch made by crushing uncooked potatoes and then harvesting the starch grains from the destroyed cells. You can buy it in health food stores or online. Although there have been no clinical trials that I know of, the anecdotal evidence (mainly internet chatter) is that a teaspoon taken in the early evening helps sleep and also leads to more vivid dreams.

If anyone likes the idea of testing this out and contributing to science, I would really appreciate it if you go to our website and sign up for a small study. It will be online and completely anonymous, but with your help we may be able to find out how useful, if at all, eating potato starch really is. If you would like to take part it is important that you read the protocol on the website before beginning, so we can be sure that the results are valid. Many thanks in advance.

Stress

Sleep deprivation leads to stress and stress leads to sleep deprivation. Along with "eat less and do more exercise," one of the more annoying bits of advice that well-intentioned people like to dish out is "try to relax." We all know we should relax, that too much stress is bad for us, and that it's spoiling our lives. The real question, beyond improving sleep quality, is what can we do about it?

I've already covered probiotics in an earlier chapter, and we know that more exercise will help. But what about other, more psychologically based techniques?

One of the tricks I find helpful when I am in an acute stressful situation, like preparing for a radio interview or doing a live TV show, is to try telling myself that what I am experiencing is not stress but excitement.

In both cases you get a rush of adrenaline, sweaty palms, agitation. Your body knows that you are not relaxed, but what it can't tell is whether you are excited or stressed.

So, repeating to yourself, "I'm really looking forward to this, which is why my pulse is racing and my hands are shaking" may help. It is certainly better than thinking, "This will be a disaster, I wish I wasn't here, help, help, help."

For more chronic stress I recommend mindfulness, a subject I've written about before but worth touching on here.

Can you change your mind?

Do you ever find yourself going for a long drive and reaching the end without being aware that you have been driving, lost as you are in your own musings?

Most of us spend our waking lives wrapped up in our own internal world. We overthink and, like overdoing anything, overthinking tends to have negative consequences. In the case of constant mental meanderings the risk is that they will lead to a negative spiral of indecisiveness, self-loathing, depression, and insomnia. One way to counter this is to make yourself more mindful.

I had been intending to try mindful meditation for some years, but never quite got around to it. Finally, three years ago I decided it was time to sort out my head. Because I wanted to measure, objectively, what effects it would have on my brain, before starting I went to see Professor Elaine Fox, then at the University of Essex, now at Oxford University.

She did a range of tests, including measuring the levels of electrical activity on the two sides of my brain while I was resting. Surprisingly enough, studies have shown that people who are prone to high levels of pessimism, neuroticism, and anxiety tend to have greater activity on the right side of their frontal cortex than on the left. This is known as cerebral asymmetry. We know it happens but we don't know why.

The results of the various tests suggested that I was a pessimist with a brain which, as Elaine kindly put it, was "on the negative side of the spectrum."

Then I went off to try mindful meditation for six weeks. Some people like joining a group, but I was running all over the place so I ended up doing it via an app.

If you want to get a flavor, try this: sit up straight in a comfortable chair, rest your hands on your thighs, close your eyes, and then for the minute or so try paying attention just to your breathing.

You don't need to speed it up or slow it down, simply pay attention to the sensation of the breath going through your nostrils, filling your chest, expanding and contracting your diaphragm. When you notice that your thoughts have drifted, which they will, gently bring your focus back to your breath.

Okay, don't read any more. Don't turn over the page. Put this book aside and give it a try. It's only a minute, what have you got to lose?

So how did it go? I predict that doing it for even a minute was tough. You probably felt uncomfortable, perhaps experienced an inner resistance, a feeling that this was a complete waste of time. This is absolutely normal, a sign that your thoughts, like wild horses, are not used to being controlled.

The Raisin Test

Another way to experience "mindfulness" is to do the raisin test. You can also do this with a square of chocolate, but I find that too distracting. Start by reading these instructions, then put the book aside. Or do it with a friend who is happy to read them out to you. Or go to our website where you can listen to me guiding you through it.

1. Take a raisin, just one, and put it in the palm of your hand. Take a close look at it. Inspect it as if you have never seen a raisin before. Pay attention to the color, the weight, the way the light reflects off its surface. Spend some time admiring it.

2. Next, pick it up with your other hand and give it a little squeeze. Roll it around in your fingers. Enjoy the texture.

---

3. Now give it a sniff. What does it smell like? What does it remind you of? Hot summer days? A glass of wine on holiday? Being young and happy? Close your eyes, enjoy the moment, breathe in those raisiny smells deeply.

4. Now put it on your tongue, but don't chew or swallow it. You can use your tongue to roll it around, but you have to resist biting. Again, close your eyes so you can properly savor it.

5. Finally, bite into it, slowly, and notice the release of flavors.

6. When you are ready, swallow it, but try to stay in the moment, simply enjoying the lingering effects of the now vanished raisin on your taste buds.

When I started practicing meditation I spent ages finding excuses not to do it. Too busy, too tired, too hungry, too stressed. The thought of Elaine Fox waiting for me at the end of the six weeks kept me on track. I also found it helpful that my wife, Clare, joined in. Even so, I spent much of the allotted time (initially ten minutes a day, building up to twenty) absorbed in my usual concerns, having to be constantly nudged back on course by the voice on my app.

The good news is that like any form of exercise it got easier to do, though I rarely managed more than a few minutes of focus at a time.

As well as sitting quietly, I tried building mindful moments into my day. Instead of just knocking back a cup of coffee, I would hold it, feel the warmth, try to focus on the muscle activity involved in bringing it to my lips, feel the warm liquid cascade down my throat, etc.

At the end of six weeks I felt noticeably calmer and my insomnia was also more under control. But what about my brain? I went back to Elaine to be retested and was amazed by the results. Whereas before my brain activity had suggested I was a pessimist, now there was a much better balance of activity between my two hemispheres, indicating a sharp reduction in negative thoughts and emotions.

But why does mindfulness have this effect? Probably because it helps strengthen your control over your own thoughts and feelings. In a study published in the journal *Social Cognitive and Affective Neuroscience*,[43] they asked fifteen volunteers to do four sets of twenty-minute classes of mindfulness. Then they used a special type of brain scan, arterial spin labeling magnetic resonance imaging, to look at their brains. The volunteers also filled in an anxiety questionnaire, before and after.

The researchers found that mindfulness reduced anxiety ratings by up to 39 percent. They also found that it increased activity in the areas of the brain that control worrying, particularly the ventromedial prefrontal cortex and the anterior cingulate gyrus. This supports the claim that mindfulness strengthens our ability to ignore negative thoughts and feelings.

Conclusion

I have become, as you can probably tell, a little bit obsessed by guts in general and the microbiome in particular. Talking to researchers and reading about the latest developments has been an incredibly exciting experience. It feels like we have come across this brand-new land, populated by strange and exotic creatures, which are only now beginning to reveal their secrets.

As with any new discovery, there are exploiters as well as explorers. Peddlers of unproven supplements and useless probiotics are well aware that there is a huge market out there, which they are keen to make money from. Food manufacturers, having sold us the alleged benefits of low-fat foods, are gearing up to produce a wide range of biome-friendly foods. Go carefully, is my advice. Unless you have a specific reason for doing so (such as IBS or to counteract antibiotic-related problems), buying probiotics may be a waste of time and money.

Instead, where possible, eat unprocessed "real" foods. Explore fermented foods. Use the recipes in this book to expand your repertoire and give your biome something to chew on. Good food should be a pleasure and it should be shared. Not just with your friends but with your Old Friends.

Keeping your biome properly fed and cared for is definitely worthwhile. If you look after all those friendly microbes then they will look after you. We are at the start of what I am convinced is a whole new way of approaching and understanding nutrition, one that could change the way we treat a wide range of diseases, from obesity to depression. This is just the beginning—there is so much more to come.

Part II

How to Reboot Your Biome:
A Two-Stage Healing Program

If you have mild IBS or problems with abdominal pain and bloating, you may want to reboot your gut bacteria. The program outlined here will benefit anyone who wants to improve their general gut health. The principle is fairly straightforward—if your symptoms improve or disappear when you remove a certain food item and then return when you reintroduce it, the symptoms are likely to be dietary. If, however, there is no change as a result of exclusion and reintroduction of a particular food, it is unlikely to be the cause of your symptoms.

The following is a simple program that many people have found useful. There are two phases: a remove and repair phase and a reintroduction phase. This is R & R for your gut. Ideally you should spend up to four weeks on the repair phase, although some people experience such rapid improvement they only need to do it for two weeks. The length of the reintroduction phase depends on whether or not you encounter problems when you reintroduce particular foods. The message is, go slowly and carefully.

Before you start

- **If you have any significant medical problems or very troublesome symptoms,** we recommend that you consult a health professional first. There may be medical reasons for your symptoms that need checking first, such as undiagnosed celiac disease, which is important to have investigated. Undiagnosed, celiac disease can cause low-grade symptoms or even no symptoms at all, but it can still lead to significant complications.

  Other conditions such as inflammatory bowel disease may require further investigation or management.

  It is important to rule out other potentially significant causes of your symptoms before embarking on dietary changes and to identify any reasons why this might not be a suitable approach for you. It may help to do the program with professional support.

  If you are underweight, suspect you have a food allergy, have other significant medical problems, or are frail or unwell, we would not advise embarking on this program.

- **Keep a detailed daily food and symptoms diary** for at least a week before you start, to help identify any pattern in relation to diet and other factors (see example on page 266 or print one via resources at cleverguts

187

.com). Ideally keep the diary going throughout the program until you identify any culprits. Although it requires an effort to maintain, a diary will help you be systematic and focused in your approach. If you see a professional, you will also have useful information available.

- **Plan ahead.** Go to a good-sized supermarket to identify what options there are to replace a missing food. This may be in the "free from" area—for example, the gluten-free versions of breads and oats. Often you can find natural substitutes, for example, rice or quinoa for gluten-containing pasta.

  If you have any significant events coming up, or holidays that will make it hard to sustain, defer your starting date.

Helpful practices to incorporate throughout

Food-related

- Cut right down on sugars, refined starchy carbohydrates, processed foods, and sweeteners, including sweetened soft drinks and juices. These are a disaster for gut bacteria and inflammation.

  We recommend you continue to keep these to a minimum during and after the program for continuing gut health.

- Avoid trans and partially hydrogenated fats. These are mainly present in spreads and some processed foods including cookies and pastries.

- Practice intermittent fasting—twelve- to fourteen-hour overnight fasts or 5:2 fasting (5 days eating normally, 2 days low-calorie fasting). Giving your gut a rest from having to constantly digest food allows the lining to regenerate and encourages the growth of "good" bacteria like *Akkermansia* (see page 56).

General strategies

- Sit down for meals and chew your food thoroughly. Try to make your mealtime relaxing! It might sound obvious, but chewing thoroughly reduces the likelihood you will overeat, because it gives your gut more time to release "I'm full" signals.

- Lower your stress levels. Staying calm soothes the gut and reduces levels of hormones such as cortisol that upset the balance of the biome.

- Improve your sleep. It is vital to get enough quality sleep, which means not eating meals late at night and committing to being in bed by 10:30 p.m. at least four nights a week.

- If you are constipated try magnesium citrate or triphala, a traditional Ayurvedic herbal treatment. You may also want to try Pia's seaweed capsules (see page 133). And drink plenty of water.

- Open the windows, get outside, start gardening. You need to let more bugs into your life.

Phase 1—REMOVE & REPAIR

Depending on how bad things are, you may need at least four weeks of R & R to give the lining of your gut a chance to repair and recover. Foods which commonly cause gut problems include gluten, dairy, eggs, soy, and coffee. You may also have particular foods that you suspect are causing a problem.

We don't recommend removing too many foods at one time, so it might be helpful to do "remove and repair" in several stages. You can always repeat the process with the less troublesome foods at a later date.

During the Remove & Repair phase try to avoid:

- Gluten and refined grains—if you remove these temporarily from your diet it will also leave more room on your plate for vegetables to boost your gut flora.

- Dairy products—particularly milk, as this contains the most lactose. The process of fermentation reduces the lactose load in yogurt and cheese. Though you may decide to remove all dairy products.

- Legumes—these contain lectin, which may contribute to bloating (reintroduce these after two weeks, particularly if you are a vegetarian, as they are a good source of protein).

- Alcohol (sorry).

- Very fibrous vegetables, such as broccoli and kale stalks, stringy beans, whole peas, and brassicas such as cabbage and brussels sprouts. These tend to be easier to digest if they are slow-cooked. Initially reduce highly prebiotic foods such as onions, garlic, and leeks. They can be reintroduced in the second phase.

Do include plenty of:

- Non-fibrous, plant-based foods—aim to fill at least half your plate with vegetables, herbs, and fruit. Include at least seven portions a day of vegetables and fruit, made up mainly of vegetables. And make them colorful. Variety is important for gut health, so try to eat twenty to thirty varieties a week.

- Good-quality proteins—these are necessary for the repair of your gut lining. You should aim for at least 1½ to 2 ounces of protein a day. Choose from fish (particularly oily fish), eggs, chicken, game, red meat (grass-fed), soy, nuts, tofu, tempeh, etc.

191

- Bitter leaf salads with vinegar or a citrus fruit–based starter—these will help to get your digestive juices flowing.

- Polyphenol-rich foods, such as herbs, spices, nuts, seeds, fruit and berries, teas, and dark chocolate (yess!).

- Phytonutrients—as in non-starchy vegetables and fruits of different colors, though restrict tropical fruits, melons, and grapes because of their high sugar content.

- Nondairy fats—such as olive oil, coconut oil, avocado, nuts, and seeds.

Phase 2—REINTRODUCTION

Once you have been through the Remove & Repair phase and are hopefully beginning to feel better, you can start to introduce new foods and reintroduce the ones you eliminated during the repair phase.

You can also start boosting your "good" bacteria by including more prebiotic and probiotic foods.

Introduce foods one at a time with a gap of at least three days between each one. The point is to try and identify the foods that are causing you problems.

Increase prebiotics

These are the foods that feed the good bacteria:

- Jerusalem artichokes, onions, leeks, garlic, fennel, asparagus, apples, chicory, bok choy

- Legumes—these can be added back after two weeks. Legumes are an important protein source for vegetarians, but reintroduce these slowly as they can cause gas and bloating.

Increase probiotics

These are foods that help you top up your "good" microbes:

- Fermented vegetables, including sauerkraut

- Live yogurts

- Kefir

- Cheese—particularly smelly cheeses like Roquefort, which are rich in bacteria

Reintroduce excluded foods

These are to be added one at a time over three days. Eat a normal portion of the suspected food. If symptoms recur after reintroduction, usually over the following few days, then withdraw it, allow a few days of recovery, and then try reintroducing something else.

Use the Daily Food & Symptoms Diary (see page 266) to track your response.

- Dairy products—start with full-fat live yogurt, cheese, and butter, and then add milk.

- Wheat/gluten—start with relatively low-gluten grains such as rye, spelt, or flaxseed. Sourdough breads are usually easier to digest as the lactic acid in the fermentation process helps neutralize the phytates in the flour. Then introduce wheat again over a few days.

- Alcohol in moderation—and with food. Choose red wine if you can.

Important considerations

If symptoms recur after completion of this plan, you can hit the reset button and repeat the whole process. However, if your symptoms are particularly troublesome and not settling as expected, we recommend you see a health professional trained in this area to give more tailored advice and perhaps investigate further.

Seek more urgent medical advice if you:

- Are passing blood and/or mucus

- Have severe and/or persistent abdominal pain

- Experience unexplained, unplanned weight loss or loss of appetite

- Have a recent change in bowel habit

- Suffer from anemia or a deficiency in important vitamins or nutrients

- Have persistent diarrhea and/or vomiting

If you suspect you suffer from a food allergy, it is very important that you see your doctor and get tested as it could be life-threatening. Fortunately, food allergies are relatively uncommon. Symptoms normally occur within minutes of being in contact with or eating the relevant substance. The typical reaction might involve a blotchy red rash, which is raised and itchy, known as urticaria. There may be vomiting and/or severe gut symptoms such as diarrhea; respiratory symptoms resulting in wheezing and difficulty breathing; itching or swelling of the lips, tongue, and palate; or, very rarely, sudden collapse.

Food allergy occurs when the body mistakenly reacts to food substances by producing an antibody, IgE, to fight it off, when eaten (or rarely even when in contact with the skin). IgE can be measured by a blood test. Once your health professional has helped identify the food substance, you can take measures to avoid it and, if needed, keep emergency medication on hand. An allergy is different from a food intolerance, which is a nonallergic hypersensitivity and is much more common. With an intolerance, the onset tends to be delayed by hours, not minutes, and the symptoms are more variable.

If you find yourself excluding food or food groups for a long period of time, we recommend that you consult a professional to ensure that the full clinical picture is considered and that you are getting a healthy balanced diet.

This approach is not suitable for children.

RECIPES

by Tanya Borowski, mBANT, IFMCP,
and Dr. Clare Bailey, GP

To start the day . . .

Standard breakfasts have become very centered around grains in the form of processed cereals and toast. Grains are a source of carbohydrates that can cause flatulence and bloating. We recommend sticking to whole grains while following our Clever Gut Diet, and eating less of them in general.

Pumpkin Porridge
(serves 2)

To put a warm glow in your belly and set you up for the day, why not try our Pumpkin Porridge? Pumpkins are high in beta-carotene, a powerful antioxidant, and in vitamins A (which supports the gut lining), C, and E. They are also rich in fiber, which boosts our microbiome diversity.

12 ounces pumpkin or butternut squash, diced and cooked
¼ cup coconut butter, or 2 tablespoons coconut oil
1 cup full-fat coconut milk
1 teaspoon vanilla bean paste or 1 teaspoon vanilla extract
Pinch of salt
½ teaspoon ground cinnamon
Handful of pomegranate seeds or blueberries, for serving

Blend all the ingredients except the fruit until you have a smooth paste. Warm the mixture gently in a pan. You may thin it with a little extra coconut milk.

Serve it warm with the pomegranate seeds.

Nutty Cinnamon Granola
(makes 10 portions)

This is one of Michael's favorites. It's a delicious combination of nuts, flaxseed, and whole grains that will keep you full for longer. It's much tastier and lower in sugar than the store-bought versions. Have it with some homemade yogurt or kefir (see page 206), and for a bit of juicy sweetness add an unpeeled diced pear.

½ cup coconut oil
½ cup honey or maple syrup (add extra 1 to 2 tablespoons if
    you have a sweet tooth)
2 teaspoons ground cinnamon

1 tablespoon vanilla extract

1 large egg white, whisked

1¾ cups rolled oats, rice flakes, or buckwheat flakes
(or a combination of all 3)

14 ounces mixed nuts (choose from walnuts, almonds,
hazelnuts, pecans, or cashews), chopped

⅓ cup ground flaxseed

1 teaspoon sea salt

Preheat the oven to 220°F. Gently heat the oil, honey, and cinnamon in a saucepan until the honey melts. Remove the pan from the heat and stir in the vanilla.

Allow the mixture to cool before mixing in the egg white.

Meanwhile, combine the oats, nuts, and flaxseed in a large bowl, then stir in the contents of the pan. Place the mixture in small clumps on a baking sheet and bake until it's golden.

This should take 1 to 1½ hours. Check it regularly and turn it once or twice. To ensure the granola is really crisp, you can then turn the oven off and leave it for a few hours or even overnight.

Allow it to cool thoroughly before storing it in an airtight container. Serve it with organic Greek yogurt and berries of your choice or a diced pear.

Creamy Cashew & Banana Breakfast Pot
(serves 2)

Bananas are a prebiotic and encourage the growth of those health-giving gut bacteria.

10 ounces raw cashews

1 medium frozen banana

¾ cup unsweetened almond milk

½ teaspoon ground cinnamon

2 teaspoons nut butter

1 teaspoon vanilla extract

Place the cashews in a bowl and cover them with water. Soak them overnight or for at least 6 hours, then drain them, place them in a blender or food processor, and blend them with all the other ingredients at a high speed, until you have a smooth paste. Pour the mixture into 2 dishes and place them in the fridge. Serve cold.

Tip: Keep some peeled, diced bananas in a ziplock bag in the freezer.

Chia Pot
(serves 1)

2 tablespoons chia seed
⅔ cup dairy-free milk of your choice (e.g., coconut,
    hazelnut, or almond milk)
½ teaspoon vanilla extract
½ teaspoon ground cinnamon
1 tablespoon berries (fresh or frozen)

Put the chia seed, milk, vanilla, and cinnamon in an airtight, or covered jar (about 12-ounce volume) and stir well. Add half the berries and stir again. Put the jar in the fridge, ideally overnight but for at least 30 minutes. The chia seed will have absorbed the liquid and plumped up. Serve with the remaining berries and one of these additional toppings:

1 to 2 tablespoons toasted coconut flakes
1 tablespoon ground almonds or flaxseed
1 to 2 tablespoons blueberries or raspberries
1 to 2 tablespoons whey protein powder (a great
    source of protein)

Healthy Gut Green Smoothie
(serves 1)

We don't like store-bought smoothies as they are usually way too sweet, but we love this homemade one. Spinach is rich in vitamins and flavonoids, which have been shown to boost beneficial bacteria in the gut, while avocado is packed with good natural fats and vitamin E.

    2 handfuls of organic spinach leaves
    1 cup water
    ½ avocado
    1 medium banana
    1 tablespoon tahini
    1 tablespoon chopped fresh ginger (optional)
    Juice of 1 lemon

Mix all the ingredients together in a blender until thick and creamy.

Kiwi & Chia Seed Smoothie
(serves 1)

Perhaps we should call this one "The Unblocker." It should certainly help move things along if you are prone to constipation.

1 kiwi
¼ medium avocado
4 tablespoons chia seed
Juice of ½ lime
1 cup water

Mix all the ingredients together in a blender until smooth.

Tanya's Leaky Gut Healing Smoothie
(serves 1)

This is one that Tanya often recommends to her patients. The collagen provides extra protein, and is particularly helpful for those with a leaky gut. A 2014 study showed consuming collagen powder can improve skin elasticity, too.[44]

¾ cup unsweetened coconut or almond milk
1 (10-ounce) package frozen spinach, or a handful of fresh
    spinach leaves
2 ounces frozen berries (e.g., raspberries or blueberries)
2 tablespoons organic collagen powder (optional)
1 teaspoon ground cinnamon

Mix all the ingredients briefly on high speed in a blender.

Nut Milk
(makes 1 cup)

Dairy foods, with the exception of homemade yogurt (if tolerated), are best avoided if you have gut problems as the casein can trigger inflammation and irritate the gut lining, while lactose can cause bloating and diarrhea. You can buy nondairy milks such as almond, coconut, or hazelnut—or make your own, following this simple recipe. It produces a luxurious, nutritious, creamy milk, plus you know exactly what's in it.

4 ounces raw cashews
⅔ cup filtered or bottled water
Small pinch of sea salt
½ teaspoon vanilla bean paste, or ¼ teaspoon vanilla extract

Soak the nuts in tap water overnight, or for at least 4 hours. Drain and rinse them. Put them in a blender with the rest of the ingredients and blend at high speed until they have broken down.

To create a smooth texture, strain the mixture into a bowl through a piece of muslin or fine sieve. Squeeze out the fluid and discard the contents of the muslin. Store the milk in an airtight container for up to 4 days. Serve it chilled or heat it gently to make a creamy hot drink.

Turmeric Latte
(serves 2)

Turmeric, like ginger, is a natural anti-inflammatory. Combined here with cardamom and ginger, it makes a warming, aromatic drink.

¼ inch fresh ginger, or ½ teaspoon ground
¾ inch fresh turmeric, or 1 teaspoon ground
1 cup plus 2 tablespoons almond or coconut milk
    (from a carton not a can)
Seeds of 2 cardamom pods
1 teaspoon honey
2 teaspoons coconut oil
Pinch of ground cinnamon

Peel and grate the ginger and turmeric. Gently heat the milk in a small pan, then add the cardamom seeds, honey, and coconut oil, whisking constantly so the milk heats through and is foamy. Pour the mixture into a cup and sprinkle with the cinnamon.

Homemade Yogurt
(makes about 1 quart)

Not only does homemade yogurt usually have a higher probiotic content than store-bought versions, it's also much tastier. And if you get into a routine, it just keeps on producing.

When fermented for 24 hours, most of the lactose is removed, which means that some people who are usually intolerant to lactose may well be able to "tolerate" it. The easiest way to make your own yogurt is probably with a yogurt maker, although there are plenty of people who do it in the traditional way, keeping it in a warm place, covered, overnight. Some store it overnight in the microwave, which acts like a large thermos flask keeping it warm.

    1 quart organic whole milk (or half whole milk
        and half light cream for a creamier texture)
    2 heaping tablespoons good-quality live organic yogurt,
        or 2 tablespoons yogurt starter
    1 quart thermos flask, or a covered bowl or a yogurt maker
    Digital thermometer (optional)
    1 quart glass container

Make sure all your equipment and containers are meticulously clean and have been sterilized in boiling water (or on a hot cycle in the dishwasher).

If using live yogurt as a starter, it helps if it is at room temperature. The containers for storing the yogurt should also ideally be at room temperature.

Put the milk in a pan and heat it gently, stirring frequently so it doesn't burn. Take it off the heat just before it comes to a boil (when it starts to bubble at the sides). Allow the milk to cool to about 85° to 104°F—it should feel just warm to the touch. (If using cream, stir it in earlier as this will also aid the cooling-off process). Then pour a cupful of milk into a bowl and stir in the starter. Add the rest of the milk and stir again so that they are well combined.

For incubation, transfer the mixture to a yogurt maker, a dry sterilized thermos flask, or a covered bowl and let it stand on the kitchen counter for 24 hours (many yogurt makers can't be set for longer than 15 hours, so just reset again when the 15 hours are up if needed). The warmer the temperature, the faster it will set (it should never be allowed to get any warmer than 115°F).

Transfer the yogurt to clean glass containers and store them in the fridge (to stop fermentation) for up to 5 days. Keep 4 tablespoons yogurt to seed the next batch within the 5 days and just keep the production line going . . .

Tip: Use goat or sheep's milk if you are sensitive to dairy. They contain a different type of casein, which you may be able to tolerate.

Milk Kefir
(makes 2 cups)

Kefir has been an enjoyable discovery. It is a fermented milk drink with a delicate flavor, and is easy to make. As with yogurt, fermentation breaks down the lactose. Kefir culture is grown from a complex ecosystem of "grains" that look a bit like tiny, soft cauliflower florets but are in fact living communities of around forty to fifty types of bacteria and yeasts. Together they produce one of the most probiotic-rich drinks available.

> 1 to 2 packages (each about ½ ounce) of kefir starter culture
>   powder, or 2 to 3 tablespoons fresh grains
> 1 quart organic whole milk
> 1 quart glass container with lid

Follow the instructions for Homemade Yogurt (page 206) for sterilizing your equipment.

If using powder, mix it into a smooth paste with a little milk in a glass measuring cup or bowl, then add this to the rest of the milk in a glass container and stir. If using grains, simply drop them into the bottom of the container, add the milk, and stir briefly. Place it in a warm spot for about 24 hours—the ideal temperature is 72° to 75°F. The kefir sets more quickly in warmer temperatures and can take up to 30 hours on a cold day. Don't stir it during the fermentation process.

It is ready when it is lightly set; you can test by scooping out a teaspoonful—it should leave a small indent in the surface. Strain it through a fine nylon sieve or muslin and place it in a covered glass container in the fridge to cool. The grains can be used again—if not using them immediately, rinse them in filtered water and freeze. In fact, if you get into the flow, you will soon have more grains than you need—give some away to create another colony!

For variations in flavor you might add a spoonful of chopped fruit, a few drops of vanilla extract, or a fruit-flavored tea bag. Kefir is delicious served with granola (page 198) and fruit.

Raspberry Chia Jam
(makes about ¾ cup)

A delicious fruity low-sugar jam which is wonderfully quick and easy to make. You can also serve it as a coulis, stirred into whole milk yogurt, or coconut-based yogurt.

1 to 1½ ounces pitted dates, finely diced, or 1 to 2 teaspoons
   maple syrup
4 ounces raspberries (frozen or fresh)
2 to 3 teaspoons chia seed (depending on how thick you like it)

Gently heat the dates in a small pan with 2 tablespoons water for about 2 minutes, stirring to form a smooth paste.

Add the raspberries and chia seed and simmer for 2 to 3 minutes. Mash the raspberries with a potato masher or the back of a spoon. The jam can be stored in an airtight container in the fridge for up to 1 week.

Green Flaxseed Bread
(makes a 2-pound loaf, 10 to 12 slices)

Flaxseed gives this bread a delicious, nutty flavor. Not only that, it is also rich in omega-3 and fiber, which your biome and your bowels will enjoy.

⅓ cup ground almonds

¾ cup plus 2 tablespoons ground flaxseed

¼ cup chia seed

¼ cup pumpkin seeds

4 large eggs

7 ounces fresh spinach (or thawed frozen)

¼ cup coconut oil or butter

1 teaspoon baking soda

2 tablespoons lemon juice

¼ cup water

1 teaspoon sea salt

Preheat the oven to 325°F. Line a loaf pan with parchment paper or grease the pan with coconut oil. Put all the ingredients in a food processor and blend until you have a smooth dough. Press it into the prepared pan and bake for 45 minutes, until it's cooked through (if you pierce it with a skewer it should come out clean). This is a fairly dense bread. Let it cool, then turn it out and cut it into slices. Store it in a ziplock bag in the fridge or in the freezer. It's delicious toasted.

Breakfast Bread
(makes a 2 pound loaf, 10 to 12 slices)

The ground almonds, flaxseed, and eggs make this a high-protein, low-grain breakfast or snack. This bread is best served warm or toasted. Try it spread with a little nut butter.

¾ cup ground almonds
2 tablespoons coconut flour
3 tablespoons ground flaxseed
1 teaspoon sea salt
1½ teaspoons baking powder
5 large eggs
2 tablespoons coconut oil
1 tablespoon maple syrup
1 tablespoon raw apple cider vinegar

Preheat the oven to 350°F. Line a loaf pan with parchment paper or grease the pan with coconut oil. Put the almonds, coconut flour, flaxseed, salt, and baking powder in a food processor and pulse until everything is combined. Then add the rest of the ingredients and pulse again to form a smooth dough. Bake for about 40 minutes, or until it's golden and cooked through (if you pierce it with a skewer it should come out clean). Let cool, then turn it out. Store it in a ziplock bag in the fridge or in the freezer, sliced.

Lunchtime

Before a meal, to get your digestive juices going, why not have a small "gin and tonic": a glass of carbonated or still water with a tablespoon of live (raw) apple cider vinegar. Ideally the vinegar should contain "the mother," strands of proteins, enzymes, and friendly bacteria that give it a murky, cobweb-like appearance and can make it look slightly congealed).

Or enjoy a salad made with a handful of bitter greens such as arugula, dandelion leaves, frisée, or chicory and Apple Cider Vinegar Dressing (page 234), which will have a similar enzyme-stimulating effect.

Buckwheat Blinis
(makes 10 to 12 medium blinis)

Despite its name, buckwheat is not related to wheat and is gluten-free. It is also a good source of minerals and antioxidants. These blinis look like a cross between a drop scone and a flat crumpet and make a brilliant savory or sweet brunch.

¾ cup buckwheat flour or another whole grain flour
1 teaspoon baking powder
Generous pinch of salt
1 large egg
⅔ cup any milk (e.g., coconut, dairy, soy, almond)

Put the flour in a mixing bowl with the baking powder and salt. Make a well in the center and add the egg and a little of the milk. Start beating the egg and milk with a fork, gradually incorporating the flour and adding more milk until you have a smooth batter. Let it stand for 20 minutes.

Lightly grease a large, flat-based frying pan or a griddle and place it over medium heat. Drop spoonfuls of the batter in the pan—you can make 3 or 4 at the same time but leave room for them to spread. Turn them over when holes appear in the surface and the top starts to firm up, 2 to 3 minutes.

Flip them over again and cook for another 1 to 2 minutes before removing them from the pan. They're delicious hot straight from the pan or you can store them in an airtight container and pop them in the toaster briefly before serving.

Tip: You could spread these with whole cream cheese or a nondairy equivalent and top them with pickled fish or smoked mackerel or salmon, a squeeze of lemon, and freshly ground black pepper.

Cashew Nut Cheese
(makes about 2 cups)

A delicious spread to try on one of our breads.

12 ounces raw cashews, soaked in water and drained
½ cup water
4 tablespoons nutritional yeast
2 tablespoons lemon juice
2 garlic cloves
1 tablespoon raw apple cider vinegar
1 tablespoon Dijon mustard
Sea salt and freshly ground black pepper to taste

Mix all the ingredients in a blender until you have a thick, creamy paste.

Tip: Use this "cheese" as an alternative to mayonnaise on a chopped boiled egg, or as a dip with vegetables or gluten-free crackers.

Walnut & Red Pepper Dip
(makes about 1 cup)

2 red bell peppers, halved and seeded
3 tablespoons extra-virgin olive oil
5 ounces walnuts, roasted

Bunch of cilantro or parsley
Salt and freshly ground black pepper to taste

Preheat the oven to 400°F. Place the bell peppers on a baking tray and drizzle the oil over them. Bake them near the top of the oven for 30 minutes, then chop them coarsely, and puree them in a blender with the remaining ingredients. Add more walnuts if you want a thicker spread. Serve it with a selection of crudités such as carrot batons, celery, cauliflower florets, or zucchini, or spread on Flaxseed, Chia & Red Pepper Crackers (page 228).

Green Seaweed Dip
(makes about 2 cups)

Seaweed is a significant part of many diets around the world, particularly in Asia, prized for its high nutritional content—it is rich in protein, fiber, and omega-3—and wonderful flavors. We are excited about finding tasty ways to incorporate more of it in our recipes.

1 yellow bell pepper
1 medium zucchini
1 (14-ounce) can beans or chickpeas, rinsed and drained
1 garlic clove, crushed
2 tablespoons olive oil
2 heaping tablespoons pesto sauce
½ pack nori sushi sheets (about ½ ounce), diced into
    ¼-inch squares

Place a wok or large pan with a lid over high heat and scorch the whole bell pepper and the zucchini for about 10 minutes, turning them occasionally. When they are charred in a few places, turn off the heat and leave them to soften in the pan with the lid on for about 5 minutes. Alternatively, char the vegetables under a hot broiler. Remove and discard the stalk, seeds, and any patches of very blackened skin. Dice the zucchini and the bell pepper. Then put them into a food processor, along with the beans, garlic, and pesto. Pulse for a minute or so, leaving a bit of texture.

Mix the nori seaweed with the vegetables, keeping aside a small handful for garnishing. Blend briefly. Pour the dip into a bowl, scatter the remaining seaweed on top, and serve it with a selection of crudités such as carrot batons, mini corn on the cob, cauliflower and/or broccoli florets, or Flaxseed, Chia & Red Pepper Crackers (page 228).

Gut-soothing Bone Broth
(serves 4 to 6)

The lining of your intestine can be damaged by all sorts of things: infections, some medications, or certain proteins. It is composed of a single layer of cells, and if the tight junctions that hold these cells together open up, you are prone to a condition called "leaky gut" or "increased intestinal permeability." Eating collagen may help. This is found in meat, gristle, skin, and bones, and boiling down bones releases the collagen into the broth.

Bone broth is hugely popular with the health and fitness crowd, even among those who don't have a leaky gut, because it also contains lots of important nutrients. It is also an ideal aid to recovery from illness.

1 medium organic chicken, or 3 pounds chicken parts (bone-in)
1 onion, chopped
3 carrots, chopped
2 celery stalks, chopped
2 to 3 zucchini, sliced
2 garlic cloves
2 tablespoons raw apple cider vinegar
2 tablespoons coconut oil
2 to 3 slices root ginger
1 teaspoon ground turmeric
Sea salt and black peppercorns

Place all the ingredients in a large saucepan with just enough water to cover them. Bring the broth to a boil, then lower the heat, put the lid on, and let it simmer, ideally for 6 to 8 hours, but for at least 2 to 3 hours, adding more water as needed.

Transfer the chicken to a platter to cool. Remove all the meat from the carcass—the meat can be used for a chicken salad (see page 235).

This broth will keep in the fridge for 3 to 4 days or can be frozen for up to 1 month. It can also be sipped as a warm drink. It is especially good with a squeeze of lemon and a little sea salt.

Creamy Cauliflower & Jerusalem Artichoke Soup

(serves 4)

Cauliflower is a good source of vitamin C and contains compounds that stimulate detoxification enzymes, while Jerusalem artichokes are full of gut-friendly inulin fiber.

2 tablespoons olive oil

1 onion, finely chopped

3 garlic cloves, coarsely chopped

½ teaspoon ground turmeric, or 1 teaspoon grated fresh

1 large head cauliflower, cut into florets

5 ounces Jerusalem artichoke, scrubbed, peeled, and sliced

1½ cups canned full-fat coconut milk

2½ cups vegetable stock

2 teaspoons tamari sauce

Freshly ground black pepper

Handful of fresh cilantro leaves, chopped

In a large saucepan, heat the oil over medium heat and gently fry the onion, garlic, and turmeric for 5 minutes. Add the cauliflower and artichoke and stir well, then pour in the coconut milk, stock, and tamari. Bring it to a boil, then immediately lower the heat, and simmer for 15 minutes, or until the vegetables are tender. Season with pepper to taste. Process the soup in a blender until it's smooth. Serve with cilantro and a slice of Green Flaxseed Bread (page 210).

Happy Gut Chicken Soup
(serves 4)

1 white onion, chopped

1 small garlic clove, chopped

2 tablespoons olive oil

2 large boneless chicken thighs, diced

3 cups water or Gut-soothing Bone Broth (page 216)

1 teaspoon chopped ginger

Juice of 1 lime

4 medium carrots, sliced

1 red bell pepper, seeded and chopped

1 yellow bell pepper, seeded and chopped

1 head broccoli, chopped

1 teaspoon chopped fresh thyme, or ½ teaspoon dried

Sea salt and freshly ground black pepper

Handful of fresh cilantro and parsley, chopped

2 teaspoons chopped fresh chives

Gently cook the onion and garlic with the chicken in the oil in a large pan until everything is golden. Then add the chicken, broth, ginger, lime juice, carrots, bell peppers, and broccoli and simmer on low heat for 60 to 90 minutes, or until the vegetables are soft and the flavors have blended. Season generously with salt and black pepper.

Add the cilantro and chives a few minutes before serving.

Carrot & Turmeric Soup
(serves 4)

Turmeric, our anti-inflammatory friend, adds color and flavor to this delicious carrot soup.

3 tablespoons olive oil

1 white onion, chopped

Pinch of sea salt

2 teaspoons ground turmeric, or ¾ inch grated fresh

1 tablespoon chopped fresh ginger

2 garlic cloves, chopped

1 pound carrots, cut into ¾-inch chunks

1½ cups Gut-soothing Bone Broth (page 216) or bouillon

Juice of 1 lime

Freshly ground black pepper

Heat the oil in a large pan over medium heat and gently cook the onion with a large pinch of salt for 5 minutes. Add the turmeric, ginger, and garlic and cook for 1 to 2 minutes, then add the carrots and stir in the broth. Bring it to a boil, then reduce the heat and let it simmer, covered, for about 25 minutes. With a hand or immersion blender, blend the soup until there are no lumps. Add the lime juice and a little more water if needed. Season with sea salt and pepper to taste.

Green Pea Soup
(serves 4)

1 pound frozen peas
2 ripe avocados
A few fresh mint leaves, chopped
2 spring onions, chopped
1 tablespoon tamari sauce or soy sauce

Cook the peas in boiling water for 3 to 4 minutes, drain and blend them with the rest of the ingredients. Season to taste.

Classic Greek Salad
(serves 2)

This old favorite makes the ideal nutritious salad—plenty of antioxidants, fiber, and vitamins (including C, A, and B_2) from the vegetables; calcium, protein, and fats from the cheese to keep you satiated and help you absorb the vitamins; and last but not least, the lovely bugs to feed that biome . . .

½ medium cucumber, seeded and cut into ¼-inch slices
2 large ripe tomatoes, or 4 medium, cut into wedges
½ small green bell pepper, seeded and finely sliced (optional)

Handful of pitted Kalamata olives

½ small red onion, finely sliced

3½ ounces good-quality feta cheese

Leaves from 1 sprig fresh oregano, finely chopped
    (or a generous pinch of dried)

2 to 3 mint leaves, finely chopped

2 tablespoons extra-virgin olive oil

1 tablespoon red wine vinegar

Sea salt and freshly ground black pepper

Spread the cucumber and tomatoes around the sides of a wide bowl. Add the bell pepper, if using, followed by the olives and onion. Place the chunk of feta on top and sprinkle the herbs over it. Drizzle generously with oil (the salad should be coated, but not drowning in it) and vinegar. Finish with a pinch of fine sea salt such as Maldon and black pepper.

Tip: Greek salads are traditionally served dressed, not tossed, with the cheese in one piece on top.

Carrot & Beet Salad
(serves 4)

Not only do beets add great flavor to a dish, they are also one of the few "superfoods" that really deserve their title. They are rich in nitrates and have even been shown to lower blood pressure.

2 tablespoons freshly squeezed orange juice

2 teaspoons freshly squeezed lemon juice

4 to 5 tablespoons olive oil

2 tablespoons tamari sauce

¼ teaspoon sea salt

12 ounces carrots, grated

12 ounces beets, peeled and grated (it is best to wear plastic gloves for this)

5 ounces pumpkin seeds

4 ounces hazelnuts

1 teaspoon coriander seed

4 ounces feta, if using dairy

Whisk the orange and lemon juices, oil, tamari, and salt to make the dressing. Toss the carrots and beets together in a salad bowl.

Put a small pan on the stove and gently fry the pumpkin seeds and hazelnuts, turning them frequently until they're golden. Throw in the coriander seed for the last minute or so. When it is cool, scatter it over the salad. Crumble the feta, if using, over the salad.

Phyto Salad Bowl
(serves 1)

This salad will help you achieve a good balance of flavor and nutrients, particularly those all-important phytonutrients. While at least three-quarters of your bowl should be plant-based, you should also ensure you get the required fats and proteins. We suggest you choose:

- *3 to 4 portions of colored vegetables (one of which can be substituted with fruit), such as*:
  1 sliced carrot
  ½ sliced bell pepper (red, orange, yellow)
  ½ sliced zucchini
  5 cherry tomatoes
  4 steamed asparagus spears
  3 to 4 artichoke or palm hearts
  ½ cup sliced radishes, sugar snap peas, or mushrooms
  Fruit: strawberries, unpeeled pear or apple, papaya, mango, grapes, pomegranate seeds, blueberries, or raspberries (about ½ cup)

- *1 to 2 cups of any of the following greens, such as*:
  Spinach, mixed leaves, arugula, kale, broccoli, chicory, cauliflower, bok choy, sprouts, Swiss chard, cabbage

- *1 to 2 portions of protein, such as*:
  2 hard-boiled eggs
  Meat: chicken, turkey, cold meat (about 3 ounces)
  Oily fish: tuna, salmon, mackerel, sardines; or white fish such as trout, cod, haddock (about 4 ounces)
  Dairy: hard cheese, halloumi, goat cheese, feta (1 to 2 ounces)

Plant protein: a generous handful of lentils, beans
(reduce both of these if you suffer from IBS or
bloating), nuts, seeds, tofu, tempeh, hummus

- *2 to 3 portions of health-boosting fats, such as*:
  ½ small avocado
  6 olives
  1 to 2 tablespoons dressing made with extra-virgin
  olive oil, sesame, walnut, or rapeseed oil
  Toasted seeds or nuts: pumpkin, pine nuts,
  sunflower, hazelnuts, cashews

- *1 to 2 portions of legumes, squash, or whole grains (optional)*:
  ¼ cup cooked quinoa, brown rice, whole barley, or
  wild red rice
  1 slice whole grain bread: millet, spelt, or rye (or
  gluten-free as required)
  ¼ cup cooked beans, lentils, or chickpeas
  ½ cup diced cooked pumpkin or butternut squash

- *And for extra flavor*:
  Fermented vegetables, such as sauerkraut or kimchi
  Pickled vegetables, such as cornichons, jalapeño peppers
  Seaweed: nori cut into strips, kelp/dulse flakes
  Fresh herbs: cilantro, mint, parsley, basil, etc.

Get those phytonutrients

Phytonutrients are the natural components of plants that keep them healthy by protecting them from disease and damage. Their antioxidant and anti-inflammatory properties also provide significant health benefits for us. Eating them helps preserve the microbial balance in the gut, keeping it in good working order.

Phytonutrients in fruit and vegetables come in a range of colors—green, yellow-orange, red, blue-purple, and white. The key is to eat a wide variety of colors, aiming for two or more of each per day.

Phyto Burst Lunchbox
(serves 1)

1. *Legumes, whole grains, or squash (optional)*:
   4 ounces butternut squash or pumpkin, cubed and roasted with a drizzle of olive oil

2. *Greens*:
   1 cup spinach leaves
   4 to 5 broccoli florets, steamed

3. *Colors*:
   ½ cup finely sliced red cabbage
   1 small-medium carrot, grated or finely sliced
   1 small red bell pepper, seeded and sliced
   4 canned artichoke hearts, drained (they taste even
       better scorched on a hot griddle)

4. *Proteins*:
   2 hard-boiled eggs, coarsely chopped
   2 tablespoons mixed seeds, toasted

5. *Health-boosting fats*:
   ½ avocado, sliced
   Dressing, e.g., Apple Cider Vinegar Dressing
       (page 234)

And for extra flavor:
   Handful of fresh cilantro, chopped
   Sea salt and freshly ground black pepper to taste

In a large bowl, or a Tupperware container if you're taking it to work, mix the cooled pumpkin, if using, with the spinach, broccoli, cabbage, carrot, bell pepper, and artichoke hearts. Add the eggs, then scatter the seeds, avocado, and cilantro leaves on top. Season with salt and pepper. Make your dressing and put it in a small screw-top jar if you're taking it to work, so you can dress your salad at lunchtime.

Flaxseed, Chia & Red Pepper Crackers
(makes about 40)

These tasty crackers go well with cheese or a dip, such as Green Seaweed Dip (page 215) or hummus (see page 230). The only trouble is they are very addictive.

1 medium red bell pepper

1 teaspoon olive oil

¾ cup plus 2 tablespoons ground flaxseed

¼ cup ground almonds

¼ cup chia seed

2 teaspoons tomato purée

Zest and juice of ½ lemon

1 tablespoon tamari sauce or soy sauce

1 teaspoon vegetable bouillon, such as Marigold, or ½ cube organic vegetable stock

Preheat the oven to 300°F. Lightly coat the bell pepper with the oil and roast it for 20 minutes, or until it's soft. Take it out of the oven, and when it has cooled, cut it in half, remove the seeds, and dice it.

Meanwhile, blend the rest of the ingredients in a food processor with ¼ cup water (or put them in a bowl and use a hand or immersion blender).

Add the bell pepper and pulse again. If the dough is too

dry and crumbly, add ½ to 1 tablespoon water, a little at a time.

Roll the dough as thin as you can without breaking it, to about ⅛ inch thick. This is easiest done between 2 sheets of parchment paper greased with coconut oil or butter. Remove the top layer of paper and place the dough on a baking sheet.

Lightly score the dough into squares and then bake for 20 to 30 minutes. Check it frequently toward the end to catch it as it starts to turn golden (you don't want it to get too brown).

At this point, remove it from the oven, turn it over and bake it for about 20 minutes or so to crisp up, checking regularly so it doesn't burn. Break it into squares, allow these to cool, and store them in a sealed container.

Tip: If you have one, use a silicone-based baking mat instead of the bottom layer of parchment paper as silicone tends to be more nonstick. If the crackers need crisping up before eating, simply pop them in the oven at 250°F for 5 minutes.

Rainbow Hummus

Basic Hummus (serves about 4)

    1 cup canned chickpeas, rinsed and drained
    Juice of ½ to 1 lemon
    1 tablespoon tahini
    1 teaspoon sea salt
    1 garlic clove, finely chopped
    5 tablespoons olive oil

Blend all the ingredients in a food processor or with a hand blender until you have a creamy paste.

Now, add some color . . .

Green Hummus (serves about 6)

Blend an extra garlic clove and a generous ½ cup cooked peas with the hummus.

Purple Hummus (serves about 6)

Blend 2 peeled, chopped roasted beets, and a few mint leaves with the hummus.

Red Hummus (serves about 6)

1 large red bell pepper, halved and seeded
Pinch of red pepper flakes (optional)

Place the red bell pepper under a hot broiler for 15 to 20 minutes, turning several times, until the skin is slightly charred in places and the flesh has softened. Coarsely chop it and blend it with the hummus, along with the red pepper flakes, if using.

Yellow Hummus (serves about 6)

1 small head cauliflower
1 tablespoon olive or coconut oil
1 extra garlic clove
2 teaspoons ground turmeric

Preheat the oven to 325°F. Remove the leaves from the cauliflower. Chop it into ¾- to 1½-inch pieces and toss them in the oil, garlic, and turmeric. Spread it out on a baking pan and bake for 15 to 20 minutes, or until it's soft and just turning golden, but not charred. Blend it with the hummus.

Dressings (1 to 2 tablespoons per serving)

Be generous with the oil in your dressings, not least because it will make salad taste better. Oil increases the absorption of some nutrients while slowing the absorption of starchy carbohydrates and sugars, helping you feel full for longer.

Anti-inflammatory Turmeric Dressing

  4 tablespoons extra-virgin olive oil
  Juice and zest of 2 lemons
  ¼ avocado
  1 garlic clove, minced
  1 tablespoon grated fresh turmeric, or 1 teaspoon of ground
  1 teaspoon honey
  Pinch of sea salt, or to taste

Blend all the ingredients in a blender. Add more avocado for a thicker consistency.

Cashew Nut Dressing

  1 tablespoon Cashew Nut Cheese (page 214)
  2 tablespoons raw apple cider vinegar

Beat the ingredients in a bowl until blended.

Simple Oil & Lemon Dressing

¾ cup extra-virgin olive oil
¼ cup lemon juice
½ teaspoon honey or maple syrup
½ teaspoon cayenne pepper, or ½ red chile, chopped
(optional)

Shake all the ingredients in a lidded jar.

Lemony Vinaigrette

Juice of ½ lemon
Zest of 1 lemon
1 tablespoon raw apple cider vinegar
1 teaspoon Dijon mustard
1 tablespoon finely chopped preserved lemon
5 tablespoons extra-virgin olive oil

Blend all the ingredients, except for the oil, in a blender.
Pour in the oil slowly to the desired consistency.

Green Vinaigrette

1 teaspoon capers, rinsed
Small handful of fresh parsley

233

Small handful of fresh basil
Small handful of fresh mint
1 tablespoon chopped fresh chives
1 garlic clove, chopped
1½ tablespoons raw apple cider vinegar
5 tablespoons extra-virgin olive oil

Blend all the ingredients in a blender.

Apple Cider Vinegar Dressing

¾ cup extra-virgin olive oil
¼ cup raw apple cider vinegar
1 tablespoon lemon juice
½ teaspoon honey or maple syrup
1 garlic clove, finely chopped

Shake all the ingredients in a lidded jar.

Hummus Dressing

2 tablespoons hummus
2 to 4 tablespoons raw apple cider vinegar
2 tablespoons nutritional yeast
Squeeze of lime
5 tablespoons extra-virgin olive oil
Salt and freshly ground black pepper

Shake all the ingredients in a lidded jar.

Main dishes

Asian Coleslaw with Leftover Chicken
(serves 4)

This brightly colored dish includes lots of gut-friendly ingredients. You can use the chicken left over from the Gut-soothing Bone Broth to make it (see page 216).

If cooking the chicken from scratch:
3 medium bone-in, skin-on chicken breasts
1 medium carrot, halved crosswise
1 medium bunch celery, halved crosswise
3 sprigs flat-leaf parsley
2 sprigs fresh thyme
2 fresh bay leaves
½ teaspoon whole black peppercorns
1 teaspoon coarse salt

4 medium carrots
1 small head white cabbage
½ small head red cabbage
1 mango, cut into slices
Couple handfuls leftover cooked chicken
Cilantro leaves
1 lime, quartered

For the dressing:
2 tablespoons tamari sauce
1 tablespoon honey
1 garlic clove, minced
Thumb-size piece of root ginger, finely chopped
2 tablespoons rice vinegar
2 tablespoons sesame oil
2 tablespoons olive oil

If cooking the chicken from scratch, put the chicken breasts in a saucepan so that they fit snugly, and cover them with ¾ inch of water. Add the vegetables and herbs. Bring to a boil, then reduce the heat and simmer for 20 to 25 minutes, skimming foam from the surface as the chicken poaches. Remove the chicken from the pan and allow it to cool, then tear it into strips. Strain the stock and reserve it to use elsewhere.

To assemble the salad, cut the carrots into fine strips with a vegetable peeler or grate them quite thickly into a large bowl. Discard the outer leaves and the cores from the cabbages and shred the leaves as finely as you can. Add them to the carrots, then mix in the mango and the cooked chicken. Make the dressing by whisking all the ingredients in a bowl. Pour it over the salad and toss everything together. Serve it with fresh cilantro leaves and a squeeze of lime.

Tip: Put the dressing in a small screw-top jar if you are taking it to work so you can dress your salad at lunchtime.

Shrimp & Seaweed in Tomato Sauce with Zucchini Noodles
(serves 4)

Welcome to the wonderful world of seaweed. Rich in omega-3 and fiber, nori is easy to use and great with shrimp.

1 medium onion, finely chopped

2 garlic cloves, chopped

3 tablespoons olive oil

2 ounces salted anchovies in oil, chopped

1 teaspoon dried thyme, or 1 tablespoon chopped fresh
  if available

2 (14-ounce) cans chopped tomatoes

12 ounces frozen shrimp, thawed

4 large zucchini, spiral sliced (if you don't have a slicer, you can
  buy zucchini noodles)

½ ounce nori sushi sheets, cut into ¼-inch squares

Gently cook the onion and garlic in 2 tablespoons of the oil over low heat for 5 to 7 minutes. Add the anchovies and thyme and stir, so they form a paste with the onions. Then add the tomatoes and simmer for another 10 minutes. Stir in the shrimp and cook them for another 5 minutes.

Bring a large pot of water to a boil so that when the sauce is ready you can quickly steam the zucchini (it will only take 1 to 2 minutes, or 1 minute if you boil it). It should be al dente and not soggy! Drain it well and drizzle the remaining oil over it. Mix the seaweed into the sauce and serve it over the zucchini noodles.

Veggie Burgers
(serves 4)

Legumes, such as chickpeas and butter beans, are an important part of the Mediterranean diet and here you can enjoy them in the form of a tasty veggie burger, bursting with fiber and goodness.

    1 onion, finely chopped
    2 carrots, grated
    2 tablespoons olive oil
    1 teaspoon ground coriander
    1 teaspoon curry powder
    1 teaspoon cumin seed
    1 (14-ounce) can chickpeas or butter beans, rinsed and
        drained
    1 large egg, whisked, or 3 tablespoons coconut milk
    Handful of fresh cilantro, chopped
    Grated zest and juice of 1 lime
    1 heaping tablespoon mixed seeds (e.g., sunflower,
        sesame, and pumpkin)
    Whole grain gluten-free flour (e.g., buckwheat) for dusting

Gently cook the onion and carrots in 1 tablespoon of the oil for 5 to 7 minutes and then stir in the coriander, curry powder, and cumin seed and continue to cook gently for a few more minutes. Using a food processor or a hand blender, briefly pulse the onion mixture with the chickpeas and the egg so they are well combined but still have some texture.

Mix in the cilantro, zest, lime juice, and seeds. Season the mixture generously with salt and pepper. Shape it into 8 medium patties, dusting your hands with flour first so that they don't stick. If you have time, leave the patties in the fridge for about 20 minutes to firm up.

When you are ready to eat, heat the remaining 1 tablespoon oil in a pan and gently cook the burgers for 10 to 12 minutes, turning them occasionally, until they are golden brown.

These are delicious with a big salad of mixed leaves, cilantro, cucumber slices, and avocado served with Lemony Vinaigrette (page 233).

Salmon & Tomato Burgers
(serves 4)

6 cherry tomatoes or grape tomatoes
½ red chile, seeded and chopped
1¾ inch fresh ginger, chopped
Bunch of fresh cilantro
2 teaspoons capers, rinsed
Zest and juice of 1 lemon
4 organic salmon fillets, skin removed

1 tablespoon whole grain gluten-free flour (e.g., buckwheat),
  plus more for dusting
2 tablespoons olive oil

Using the lowest setting on your hand blender or food processor so that you keep some texture, briefly mix the tomatoes with the chile, ginger, cilantro, capers, lemon zest, and half the lemon juice.

Dice the salmon and stir it into the mixture, then pulse again, but only very briefly so that the salmon is just flaked, not mushy. Add 1 tablespoon flour to bind the mixture. Shape it into 8 smallish patties, dusting your hands with flour first so that they don't stick. Place the patties on a plate, cover them with plastic wrap, and leave them in the fridge to firm up for 20 minutes.

Heat the oil in a large, flat-based pan. Brown the patties on both sides, then reduce the heat and fry them gently for 8 to 10 minutes, or until they're cooked through.

You might serve them with a large salad or greens, and a couple of spoonfuls of cooked quinoa.

Kashmiri Chicken Curry
(serves 4)

The dark chicken thigh meat is higher in both vitamins A and D (essential for your gut health and immune function) than the white meat.

1 tablespoon coconut oil

1 pound skinless, bone-in chicken thighs

1 large onion, sliced

2 garlic cloves, finely chopped

1 green chile, thinly sliced

¾ inch fresh ginger, grated

1 teaspoon ground coriander, or 6 to 7 seed pods

1 teaspoon ground cardamom

1 teaspoon ground turmeric

4 ounces flaked almonds

½ cup chicken stock or bouillon

1 cup full-fat Greek yogurt

Bunch of fresh cilantro, chopped

Sea salt and freshly ground black pepper

Heat the oil in a large saucepan and brown the chicken pieces. Transfer them to a plate and set them aside. Gently cook the onion, garlic, chile, and ginger in the same pan for 5 to 7 minutes, or until they start to soften. Add the spices and cook for another 5 minutes, then add the almonds and the chicken. Pour in the stock and the yogurt and stir well. Season with salt and black pepper to taste.

Cover the pan with a lid and simmer for 40 minutes over a gentle heat, stirring occasionally and adding more water if needed. Alternatively, cook the curry in a casserole in an oven preheated to 300°F. Stir in the cilantro before serving.

This curry goes well with brown basmati rice or Cauliflower "Rice" (page 256) and steamed greens.

Goan Fish Curry with Seaweed
(serves 4)

This aromatic curry is packed with health-boosting nutrients, including seaweed. Cod is rich in selenium, iodine, and choline, while turmeric, garlic, and ginger are known for their antimicrobial properties—Indians have been using them for centuries to reduce the risk of gut infections.

2 tablespoons coconut oil

1 teaspoon mustard seeds

2 teaspoons ground coriander

1 teaspoon ground cumin

½ teaspoon turmeric

½ teaspoon garam masala

1 medium onion, coarsely chopped

¾ inch fresh ginger, coarsely chopped

6 garlic cloves, coarsely chopped

1 mild or medium red chile, seeded and chopped

1 tablespoon raw apple cider vinegar

1½ cups full-fat coconut milk

1 large tomato, finely diced

1 pound firm white fish (e.g., cod, pollock, haddock, or hake), cut into large chunks

½ ounce nori sushi sheets

Handful of fresh cilantro, plus more for garnish

For a vegetarian option:

10 ounces sweet potato or butternut squash, peeled, cut into
chunks, and cooked

10 ounces canned chickpeas, rinsed and drained

Heat the oil in a large saucepan and fry the spices for 1 to 2 minutes. Blend the onion, ginger, garlic, and chile with the vinegar to make a paste. Add the paste to the pan and cook for 2 minutes, until you see the oil separate. Add the coconut milk and the tomato and bring to a boil.

Add the fish and simmer until it is cooked through, 10 to 12 minutes. If doing the veggie option, add the sweet potato and chickpeas and gently heat them through for a few minutes. Chop a 1½-inch strip off the pack of nori seaweed, then cut the strip into ⅛-inch-wide (very thin) pieces and stir them into the curry.

For a fuller seaweed taste, add another, larger strip, 1 to 1½ inches wide. Check the seasoning—it may be salty enough with the seaweed.

Finally, stir in the cilantro, saving a few leaves for garnish.

Serve with Cauliflower "Rice" (page 256) or a couple of spoonfuls of brown basmati rice and a green vegetable.

Chicken Goujons
(serves 4)

You will be glad to hear that these taste nothing like the sad little nuggets you buy at takeout restaurants. The browner meat of the chicken thighs is juicier and more flavorsome than the breast. It also contains more nutrients.

- 4 boneless chicken thighs
- 1 teaspoon dried oregano
- 1 teaspoon garlic powder
- 1 teaspoon onion powder
- ½ teaspoon sea salt
- ½ cup ground almonds
- 1 large egg, beaten
- 2 tablespoons olive oil or coconut oil

Cut the chicken into ¾-inch-wide strips. In a small bowl, combine the oregano, garlic powder, onion powder, salt, and almonds. Dip the chicken pieces in the egg, then coat them evenly with the spice mixture.

Heat the oil in a large pan and fry the chicken pieces, turning them occasionally until they're golden and cooked through. Serve them with some homemade hummus (page 230), sliced avocado, and a large green salad.

Harissa & Beet Salmon
(serves 2)

Beets and salmon work surprisingly well together. You will find za'atar and harissa paste in most big supermarkets.

2 organic salmon fillets

1 tablespoon za'atar

Sea salt and freshly ground black pepper

8 ounces beets

2 medium sweet potatoes

1 fennel bulb

1 teaspoon ground cumin

4 tablespoons olive oil

1 carrot

Juice of 1 lime

2 tablespoons harissa paste

1 tablespoon sliced or chopped almonds, toasted

Preheat the oven to 325°F. Rub the salmon with the za'atar, a pinch of salt, and a grind of pepper and put it aside.

Peel the beets, halve or quarter them if large, and cut them into very thin slices. Peel the sweet potatoes, quarter them lengthwise, and dice them into ¾-inch chunks. Trim and quarter the fennel bulb and put it in a medium to large baking dish, along with the beets and sweet potatoes. Scatter the cumin over it, season with salt and pepper, and drizzle 1 tablespoon of the oil over the surface. Place the dish

245

on the middle rack of the oven for around 25 minutes, or until everything is soft, stirring once or twice.

Meanwhile, grate the carrot into a bowl and mix it with half the lime juice. In another bowl, whisk 2 tablespoons of the oil, the harissa, the rest of the lime juice, and a pinch of salt. When the vegetables are ready, remove them from the oven, pour the dressing over them, add the carrot and toss everything together. Place a frying pan over medium heat and fry the salmon in the remaining 1 tablespoon oil for 3 minutes, skin side down. Then flip them over and cook them on the other 3 sides for a minute each.

Serve the salmon on top of the baked vegetables, with the almonds scattered over it.

Mackerel or Cod in Salsa Verde
(serves 2)

Oily mackerel is the perfect foil for this feisty-flavored sauce—and a favorite of Michael's. It's also a great source of omega-3 and vitamins B_{12} and D.

2 mackerel or cod fillets
Green Vinaigrette (page 233)

Preheat the oven to 350°F. Place the fish in a baking dish lined with parchment paper, rub a good tablespoonful of the vinaigrette over it, and bake for 20 minutes.

Serve with more of the vinaigrette, some roasted veggies, and seasonal greens.

Turkey Burgers
(serves 4)

Turkey is a high-quality protein, which helps you feel full for longer. Frozen spinach is just as nutritious as fresh.

1 onion, chopped
2 garlic cloves, crushed
2 teaspoons dried oregano
8 large basil leaves
3 handfuls of baby spinach
Zest of 1 lemon
½ teaspoon sea salt
Freshly ground black pepper
3 tablespoons extra-virgin olive oil
1 pound ground turkey

Mix the onion, garlic, oregano, basil, spinach, lemon zest, salt, and pepper in a food processor with 1 tablespoon of the oil, just briefly to retain some texture. Place the mixture in a large bowl and combine it with the ground turkey, using either your hands or a rubber spatula. Shape the mixture into 8 patties and pop them in the fridge for at least 20 minutes to firm up. Place a griddle or a frying pan over medium-high heat and fry the patties in the remaining 2 tablespoons oil until they've browned—they'll need approximately 5 minutes on each side. Serve them with a large salad, some hummus (page 230), and grilled zucchini.

Beef Goulash
(serves 4)

Like all red meats, beef is loaded with iron, in which many people, particularly women, are chronically deficient. It's a high-quality protein and contains all eight essential amino acids. Do buy good-quality grass-fed if you can.

4 tablespoons olive oil

1 large white onion, chopped

2 large carrots, cut into small sticks

1 large green bell pepper, seeded and sliced

3 garlic cloves, crushed

1 pound braising beef (such as top round or chuck), diced

1 tablespoon paprika

3 tablespoons tomato purée

3 bay leaves

1½ cups Gut-soothing Bone Broth (page 216)
   or organic beef stock

1 (14-ounce) can diced tomatoes

1 tablespoon raw apple cider vinegar

Preheat the oven to 325°F. Heat 2 tablespoons of the oil in a large casserole with a tight-fitting lid and fry the onions gently for 5 to 7 minutes. Add the carrots, bell pepper, and garlic and cook for few more minutes.

Place the remaining 2 tablespoons oil in another pan over high heat and brown the meat on all sides. Season it and add it to the vegetables in the casserole, along with the paprika, tomato puree, and bay leaves. Pour the broth into the pan you used for the meat and stir for a minute or so, scraping the bottom, to incorporate all the juices from the meat, then add it to the casserole, along with the tomatoes and vinegar. Bring the goulash to a simmer, then cover it and place it in the middle of the oven for 2½ to 3 hours, taking it out occasionally to give it a stir, and adding more water if it is drying out. Remove and discard the bay leaves.

Serve it by itself with a dollop of full-fat organic Greek yogurt or a nondairy equivalent, or with a generous serving of green vegetables and a few reheated new potatoes (as these contain some resistant starch).

Caribbean Coconut & Vegetable Curry
(serves 6)

A colorful and filling vegetarian dish bursting with flavor. It looks like a lot of ingredients, but they are easy to put together and you just stick it in the oven. Adding black pepper significantly enhances the benefits of turmeric.

4 tablespoons coconut oil

1 large onion, diced

1 teaspoon each of ground coriander, cumin, and turmeric

½ teaspoon ground cinnamon, or 1 cinnamon stick

2 garlic cloves, chopped

1¾ to 2 inch fresh ginger, finely chopped

1 chile, seeded and finely chopped

1¾ cups canned full-fat coconut milk

⅔ cup vegetable stock

2 limes: 1 for juice and 1 cut in wedges

4 to 5 large pitted dates, chopped (or 2 teaspoons maple
   syrup)

14 ounces butternut squash, seeded and diced into 1-inch
   pieces

2 red bell peppers, seeded and cut into strips

1 (14-ounce) can black-eyed peas, rinsed and drained
   (optional)

10 ounces cherry tomatoes

7 ounces kale, chopped and thick stalks removed

Sea salt and freshly ground black pepper

Bunch of fresh cilantro, chopped

4 ounces cashews

Preheat the oven to 350°F. In a large casserole with a tight-fitting lid, heat the oil and fry the onion over medium heat for 5 to 7 minutes, or until it's golden. Then add the coriander, cumin, turmeric, cinnamon, garlic, ginger, and chile and fry them for 2 to 3 minutes. Next pour in the coconut milk, stock, and lime juice, along with the dates, butternut squash, bell peppers, black-eyed peas, and tomatoes. Cover the casserole and put it in the oven.

After 20 to 25 minutes, remove the casserole from the oven and stir in the kale. Return it to the oven for a few more minutes until the kale is cooked. Season with salt and plenty of black pepper. Stir in some of the cilantro and scatter the rest on top along with a sprinkling of cashews, and serve with the lime wedges.

> **Tip:** For extra flavor, use whole spice seeds and grind them in a mortar and pestle before cooking. For convenience, you can buy chopped butternut squash in the market. Skip the black-eyed peas if you're avoiding legumes.

Lamb & Sweet Potato Stew
(serves 5 to 6)

Lamb is a succulent outdoor-reared meat, and makes a great stew. Slow-cooked food tends to be easier to digest.

1¾ pounds stewing lamb, cubed
½ teaspoon each of ground cinnamon, nutmeg, cloves, and
   ginger, or 2 teaspoons mixed spice
3 tablespoons olive oil
2 large red onions, sliced
4 bacon strips
3 bay leaves

2 cups Gut-soothing Bone Broth (page 216) or organic beef
   stock
6 celery stalks, diced into ¼- to ¾-inch pieces
4 medium sweet potatoes, diced

Preheat the oven to 325°F. Place the lamb in a bowl and toss it with the spices and some seasoning. Marinate overnight or at least for a couple of hours.

Put the oil in a large casserole with a tight-fitting lid and sauté the onions for 5 to 7 minutes, or until they start to turn golden. In a nonstick saucepan, sear the meat over high heat, then pour it into the casserole with any juices.

Add the bacon, bay leaves, and broth. Bring the stew to a simmer, then place it in the oven for 2 to 3 hours, check occasionally and add more water if it starts to dry out.

Halfway through the cooking time, add the celery and sweet potatoes. Remove and discard the bay leaves. Serve the stew with quinoa and an enzyme-stimulating green salad (see page 212).

Creamy Cashew Mushrooms
(serves 2)

Mushrooms are an underrated food source. They are high in fiber, rich in B vitamins, selenium, and copper, and also very low in calories. Leaving them out in the sun for an hour or two will significantly boost their vitamin D levels.

1 tablespoon coconut oil or butter
1 large onion, diced
1 large garlic clove, crushed
12 ounces chestnut or mixed exotic mushrooms, sliced
½ teaspoon each of red pepper flakes, dried thyme, crushed
    pink peppercorns, and paprika
1 to 1½ ounces cashews
½ mushroom stock cube, or 1 vegetable stock cube
⅔ cup coconut cream
Juice of ½ lemon
Sea salt and freshly ground black pepper
Small bunch of fresh parsley, chopped, for garnish

In a medium skillet, heat the oil over medium heat and gently cook the onion for 5 to 7 minutes, then add the garlic, mushrooms, red pepper flakes, thyme, peppercorns, and paprika.

Add the cashews and cook for a few more minutes. Crumble in the stock cube, then stir in the coconut cream and lemon juice. Season with salt and a generous amount of black pepper. Simmer for a couple of minutes until everything melds together into a delicious, aromatic stew. Garnish with parsley.

Serve with sliced spring greens or zucchini. If you're hungry, add 1 to 2 tablespoons cooked brown basmati rice per person. Ideally the rice should be cooked, cooled for 12 hours, and reheated to boost resistant starch.

Baked Rainbow Ratatouille
(serves 4)

This rainbow-colored ratatouille is bursting with a whole range of phytonutrients.

For the tomato sauce:
2 tablespoons olive oil
1 medium onion, sliced
2 garlic cloves, chopped
Bunch of fresh basil leaves, chopped
1 tablespoon chopped fresh oregano leaves, or 1 teaspoon
    dried
6 medium tomatoes, chopped
1 (14-ounce) can chopped organic tomatoes
1 tablespoon balsamic vinegar
Sea salt and freshly ground black pepper

1 cup tomato sauce
4 beets
4 sweet potatoes
3 red onions
2 zucchini
1 fennel bulb
1 small pumpkin, or ½ butternut squash, seeded
    and quartered
2 yellow bell peppers
1 teaspoon sea salt

Freshly ground black pepper

2 tablespoons olive oil

To make the tomato sauce, heat the oil in a saucepan over medium heat and fry the onion gently for 6 to 7 minutes until it's soft and golden. Stir in the garlic, basil, and oregano, followed by the fresh and canned tomatoes and vinegar. Season the sauce with a pinch of salt and black pepper and let it simmer for 15 to 20 minutes. Blend it briefly and set it aside (it will keep in the fridge for about 5 days).

Preheat the oven to 375°F. Liberally cover the bottom of a large baking dish with the homemade tomato sauce (you only need about half of it for this recipe). Cut all the vegetables into ¼-inch slices, except the zucchini and bell peppers, which need to be thicker (more like ¾ inch). Starting from the outer edge of the dish, arrange the vegetables by color: slices of beet, then sweet potato, onion, zucchini, and so on until you fill it. Season with the salt and black pepper and drizzle the oil over the surface. Bake for 30 to 40 minutes.

This works well with some steamed kale or a large green salad and avocado, dressed with Green Vinaigrette (page 233).

Cauliflower "Rice"
(serves 2)

This is a low-carb alternative to rice, with far more nutrients. It's a great way of getting more cauliflower into your diet.

½ head cauliflower
2 tablespoons pine nuts
½ teaspoon sea salt
Freshly ground black pepper
Juice of ½ lemon
2 teaspoons tahini
½ teaspoon cumin seed
½ teaspoon ground turmeric
1½ teaspoons olive oil

Preheat the oven to 400°F. Either grate the cauliflower or cut it into florets and pulse it in a food processor until it resembles grains of rice. Toss it in a bowl with the rest of the ingredients and then spread it out in a thin, even layer in a baking pan. Roast for 10 to 12 minutes, turning it halfway through—this dries the "rice" out, giving it a fluffy texture.

Purple Sauerkraut
(makes about 2 cups)

Sauerkraut is one of the easiest fermented foods to make and is packed full of probiotic bacteria.

7 ounces beets, grated (use carrots if you don't like beets)
12 ounces red cabbage, very finely sliced
½ small apple, peeled, cored, and finely diced
½ teaspoon caraway seeds
1 teaspoon fennel seeds
1 teaspoon coriander seeds
2 teaspoons sea salt

Wear rubber gloves to avoid staining your hands red. Put the beets in a large bowl along with the cabbage and apple. Add the seeds and salt and massage them well into the vegetables until they start to exude water. Firmly crush the vegetables with your hands or a blunt object like a pestle or the end of a rolling pin.

Pack the mixture into a sterilized resealable 2-cup glass jar, leaving about ¾-inch headspace to allow the mixture to bubble and fizz—remember it's alive!

You need to push the vegetables down hard so that they are totally submerged in their juices. You could insert a weight to hold them down (a boiled beach pebble works well, or a chunk of cabbage stalk).

Leave the sauerkraut at room temperature for up to

3 weeks, but for at least 3 days. The longer you leave it to ferment, the more sour and distinctive its flavor.

Check and taste it regularly. Open the jar daily for the first 2 to 3 days to release the carbon dioxide, and keep checking that the vegetables are fully submerged in the brine. Continue to check your ferment regularly and push the contents below the surface of the brine if needed. If you find it's drying out, add ½ teaspoon salt to ½ cup filtered water, and use this to top it off.

Don't be alarmed if yeasts form on the surface of the sauerkraut; you can scrape these off. When you are ready to eat it, remove any discolored vegetables from the top. You can keep it in the fridge for several months.

Tip: It is important to use filtered water because most of the chlorine will have been removed—chlorine kills the bacteria needed for fermentation.

Treats

Chocolate Eggplant Brownies
(makes 12 small squares)

Strange as it may sound, the eggplant works brilliantly with the dark, flavonoid-rich chocolate. Truly yummy.

1 medium eggplant (about 7 ounces), peeled and diced
5 ounces dark chocolate (minimum 70% cocoa solids), broken
    into pieces
¼ cup coconut oil
2 ounces soft pitted dates, diced
½ teaspoon salt
3 large eggs, beaten
1 teaspoon baking powder
3½ ounces ground almonds

Preheat the oven to 325°F. Line a medium baking pan with parchment paper. Steam the eggplant for 15 minutes until it's soft (or microwave it in less time). Put it in a medium mixing bowl and stir in the chocolate and oil. The warm eggplant will melt the chocolate and oil. Add the dates and salt. Using a hand blender or a food processor, mix the batter until it's smooth. By now it should be cool enough

259

to add the eggs and baking powder. Mix again for another minute or so and then mix in the almonds. Spread the mixture in the pan and bake for about 20 minutes. It is cooked when a knife inserted into the center comes out clean.

Serve the brownies with Raspberry Chia Jam (page 209) and/or full-fat organic Greek yogurt.

Tip: Alternatively, to make cupcakes, divide the mixture among a 12-well muffin pan lined with cupcake liners and bake for 15 to 20 minutes.

Quick Baked Apple Slices
(serves 2)

A quick, nutritious go-to dessert which takes a few minutes to prepare—it goes in the oven just before you start your meal and is ready in 20 minutes.

  3 large sweet eating apples
  1 tablespoon coconut oil, melted, plus more for greasing
  1 heaping teaspoon ground cinnamon
  2 tablespoons pistachios

Preheat the oven to 325°F. Lightly grease the bottom of a baking dish with oil. Core the apples, quarter them, and cut each quarter into 2 to 3 wedges, leaving the skin on. Place the wedges in a slightly overlapping layer in the baking dish, drizzle the oil over them, and sprinkle the cinnamon on top.

Bake the apples for 10 minutes, then scatter the pistachios over them and bake for another 5 to 10 minutes. They are ready when they start to brown around the edges. Serve them as they are, or with a generous dollop of full-fat organic Greek yogurt.

PHASE 1—REMOVE & REPAIR MEAL PLANNER

This phase is gluten- and dairy-free, very low in grains and legumes (except hummus), and two servings of fruit a day. Plants are center stage—think variety and color. Avoid snacking between meals and try to fast overnight for a good 12 hours.

	Breakfast
SUN	2 eggs scrambled with wilted spinach and tomatoes. Slice of *Green Flaxseed Bread* spread with coconut oil
MON	*Leaky Gut Healing Smoothie*
TUE	*Nutty Cinnamon Granola* with *Nut Milk** and a handful of berries
WED	*Pumpkin Porridge* and a handful of blueberries
THU	2 slices *Breakfast Bread* with *Rainbow Hummus*, smoked salmon, and red pepper flakes
FRI	*Chia Pot* with 1 tablespoon each of blueberries and ground almonds
SAT	*Healthy Gut Green Smoothie* with 1 slice *Breakfast Bread* and 1 tablespoon of almond or cashew nut butter

Lunch	Dinner
Enzyme-stimulating Green Salad, followed by *Carrot & Turmeric Soup* with *Flaxseed, Chia & Red Pepper Crackers* with *Rainbow Hummus*	*Turkey Burgers* with sweet potato wedges, green leaf salad, and *Anti-inflammatory Turmeric Dressing*
Left-over *Turkey Burgers* with *Carrot & Beet Salad*	*Creamy Cashew Mushrooms* with steamed broccoli and kale with red pepper flakes
Enzyme-stimulating Green Salad followed by *Happy Gut Chicken Soup*	*Salmon & Tomato Burgers* with broccoli and *Hummus Dressing*
Phyto Salad Bowl with *Flaxseed, Chia & Red Pepper Crackers*	*Kashmiri Chicken Curry* with *Cauliflower "Rice"*
Enzyme-stimulating Green Salad followed by *Shrimp & Seaweed in Tomato Sauce* with *Zucchini Noodles*	*Baked Rainbow Ratatouille* with green leaf salad and *Lemony Vinaigrette*
Enzyme-stimulating Green Salad followed by leftover *Rainbow Ratatouille* with *Rainbow Hummus* and 1 slice *Green Flaxseed Bread*	*Cod in Salsa Verde* with steamed green beans and baby new potatoes
Phyto Salad Bowl with *Flaxseed, Chia & Red Pepper Crackers*	*Enzyme-stimulating Green Salad* followed by *Beef Goulash* with wilted greens or kale

* Nut Milk—either homemade as per recipe (page 204) or store-bought coconut (carton not can), almond, hemp, or hazelnut

PHASE 2—REINTRODUCTION MEAL PLANNER

Include more prebiotic plants: asparagus, bananas, Jerusalem artichokes, leeks, onions, bok choy, and legumes. Add probiotic foods, including fermented foods: sauerkraut, yogurt, and kefir. Add a few more grains, but still do your best to avoid wheat—go for rye, spelt, or a good sourdough that has been fermented.

	Breakfast
SUN	*Chia Pot* with 1 tablespoon raspberries and a small glass of *Kefir*
MON	*Nutty Cinnamon Granola* with *Homemade Yogurt* and a handful of blueberries
TUE	2 poached or scrambled eggs, a handful of washed spinach leaves, and 6 baby tomatoes. A slice of toasted rye bread and butter
WED	*Creamy Cashew & Banana Breakfast Pot* and a slice *Breakfast Bread* with *Raspberry Chia Jam*
THU	*Kiwi & Chia Seed Smoothie* and a slice *Breakfast Bread* with nut butter and a handful of blueberries
FRI	*Homemade Yogurt* with 2 tablespoons of ground flaxseed, a tablespoon of blueberries, and half a banana
SAT	2 boiled eggs with 4 to 6 steamed asparagus spears and a slice of toasted *Green Flaxseed Bread* or sourdough

Lunch	Dinner
Classic Greek Salad and *Flaxseed, Chia & Red Pepper Crackers*	Roast chicken and a variety of roasted vegetables. *Quick Baked Apple Slices*
Asian Coleslaw with *Leftover Chicken* (using previous night's roast)	*Harissa & Beet Salmon* with steamed asparagus and broccoli drizzled with olive oil
Enzyme-stimulating Green Salad followed by *Creamy Cauliflower & Jerusalem Artichoke Soup* with toasted *Green Flaxseed Bread*, half an avocado, and drizzled olive oil	*Turkey Burgers* with multicolored salad, *Lemony Vinaigrette*, and a tablespoon *Purple Sauerkraut*
Phyto Burst Lunchbox with some *Purple Sauerkraut*	*Goan Fish Curry with Seaweed* and brown basmati rice
Enzyme-stimulating Green Salad followed by 2 slices toasted *Green Flaxseed Bread* with canned sardines, tomato, and watercress	*Veggie Burgers* with sweet potato wedges and 3 to 4-color salad with *Anti-inflammatory Turmeric Dressing*
Enzyme-stimulating Green Salad followed by leftover *Veggie Burgers* with crudités* and *Rainbow Hummus*	*Chicken Goujons* with *Walnut & Red Pepper Dip*, brown rice, and *Carrot & Beet Salad*
Phyto Salad Bowl	*Lamb & Sweet Potato Stew* with steamed greens or kale

*crudités = chopped pieces of cucumber, peppers, carrots, asparagus, zucchini, butter lettuce, radishes, steamed broccoli, or cauliflower florets

CLEVER GUT DAILY FOOD & SYMPTOMS DIARY

Meal	Time	Food & Drink (content & quantity)
Breakfast		
Snack?		
Lunch		
Snack?		
Dinner		
Snack?		

Date: _____

Symptoms e.g., bloating, abdominal pain, nausea, sickness, diarrhea, brain fog, irritability, headache	Symptom time & duration	Other factors including stress, poor sleep, exercise, illness, medicines, and remedies

Foods high in resistant starch

Resistant starch is a form of starch that is resistant to being broken down in your small intestine. Instead of causing your blood sugars to spike, it acts more like fiber, reaching the colon largely intact. It is a valuable source of nutrients for the "good" bacteria in your gut. A diet rich in resistant starch has been linked to reduced gut inflammation and reduced risk of type 2 diabetes and obesity.

Although it acts in a similar way to fiber, it is not always found in the same foods. Breakfast cereals like All-Bran, which have decent levels of fiber, do not contain any resistant starch.

A word of warning: if you are currently on a typical Western diet, low in fiber, you should not suddenly hit your gut with a massive dose of resistant starch. Otherwise you could find yourself becoming uncomfortably bloated and gassy. Ease into it. You can afford to go up to around 1 to 1½ ounces of resistant starch a day, but I wouldn't go much higher. Our menus contain foods with moderate levels of resistant starch.

Below is a list of foods with the highest to the lowest levels of resistant starch, given as grams per 100 grams (3.5 ounces) of food. You will see from this list that there is a striking difference between unripe and ripe bananas.

You will also notice something that appears to be very confusing about resistant starch: while some foods become *more* resistant when cooked and cooled, others become less so. Potatoes and rice, for example, more than double their levels of resistant starch when cooked and cooled. Oats, on the other hand, have very high levels when raw (11 grams) but these fall to almost nothing (0.3 grams) when cooked. I occasionally have raw oats with yogurt and berries for breakfast.

Potato starch behaves quite differently from fresh potatoes

in that it has far higher levels of resistant starch when raw. Levels drop to almost zero when it is cooked. You can buy it from health food stores or over the internet as a white powder. It is totally bland and incredibly cheap.

Potato starch is also the odd one out on this list because it is highly processed. I wouldn't normally recommend processed foods but I am interested in the potential link between potato starch and insomnia. I have started taking a teaspoon mixed with kefir, yogurt, or half a glass of milk before bed.

You can find a longer list of foods and their resistant starch levels at http://freetheanimal.com/wp-content/uploads/2013/08/Resistant-Starch-in-Foods.pdf.

The following are averages, in grams of resistant starch per 100g (4 ounces) of food, based on different studies. Because the research is new there are no figures for what happens to rice or potatoes that are cooked, cooled, and then reheated.

High

Potato starch	72	Cashews	13
Unripe bananas	19	Oats, rolled, uncooked	11

Medium

Peas, cooked	6.7	Hummus	4.1
Lentils, cooked	6.6	Baked beans	3.6
Potatoes, cooked & cooled	5.8	Plantain, cooked	3.5
Brown rice, cooked & cooled	5.5	Ripe banana	3.2
Chestnuts	4.9	Kidney beans, canned	2.1
Rye bread	4.3	Sourdough bread	2.1
Peanuts	4.2		

Low

Puffed rice crackers	0.8	Croissant	0.4
Baked potatoes	0.6		

Which probiotics work and for what

The following information is taken from Medline Plus, part of the US National Library of Medicine. It is a reliable source of the latest information.

Are probiotics safe?
In healthy people, yes. But you are advised not to take them if you are pregnant, have recently had surgery, or have a faulty immune system.

The two most studied strains are *Lactobacillus* and *Bifidobacteria*, which are found in fermented foods like yogurt, kefir, and cheese. But it is more complicated than that because there are so many different species of each. Just because one species of *Lactobacillus* might help prevent diarrhea, it doesn't mean that another will.

How effective are they?
The Natural Medicines Comprehensive Database rates treatments as: Effective, Likely Effective, Possibly Effective, Possibly Ineffective, Likely Ineffective, Ineffective, and Insufficient Evidence to Rate. None of the probiotics you can buy in capsule form has sufficient studies behind it to fall into the "Effective" category, while a number fall into the "Likely Ineffective" or "Ineffective" category.

The following list only includes those considered "Likely Effective" or "Possibly Effective."

Bifidobacteria

Constipation. *Bifidobacterium longum*, whether in the form of capsules or from fermented foods, can increase bowel movements in constipated adults. This strain also seems to help prevent the flu in elderly people.

Irritable bowel syndrome (IBS). Taking VSL#3, a product containing *Bifidobacterium, Lactobacillus,* and *Streptococcus* may decrease bloating in people with IBS. It is the probiotic that my experts favored.

Lung infections. Taking HOWARU Protect, which contains *Lactobacillus acidophilus* and *Bifidobacterium,* may help reduce and shorten symptoms of fever, cough, and runny nose.

Diarrhea in children caused by rotavirus. Taking *Bifidobacterium bifidum* seems to help prevent rotaviral diarrhea when used with other bacteria such as *Streptococcus thermophilus* or *Bifidobacterium* Bb12.

Traveler's diarrhea. Taking *Bifidobacterium* may help prevent traveler's diarrhea when used with other bacteria such as *Lactobacillus acidophilus* or *Lactobacillus bulgaricus.*

Lactobacillus

Diarrhea in children caused by rotavirus. This is most likely to be effective if you use at least ten billion colony-forming units (CFUs—see page 273) for the first forty-eight hours after diarrhea starts.

Hay fever. Taking at least two billion CFUs of *Lactobacillus paracasei* daily for five weeks may improve quality of life for people with grass pollen allergy.

Preventing diarrhea caused by antibiotics. *Lactobacillus* seems to reduce the risk of diarrhea caused by antibiotics. Giving children *Lactobacillus* GG (Culturelle) along with antibiotics is a good idea.

Eczema (atopic dermatitis). *Lactobacillus* GG may reduce symptoms of eczema in infants who are allergic to cow's milk. *Lactobacillus sakei, Lactobacillus plantarum,* and a combination of freeze-dried *Lactobacillus rhamnosus* and *Lactobacillus reuteri* also seem to reduce eczema symptoms in children under thirteen. But *Lactobacillus paracasei* doesn't seem to help eczema.

Preventing diarrhea due to cancer treatment (chemotherapy). There is some evidence that patients with cancer of the colon or rectum have less severe diarrhea and have shorter hospital stays if they take *Lactobacillus rhamnosus* and *Lactobacillus* GG (Culturelle).

Irritable bowel syndrome (IBS). *Lactobacillus acidophilus* can improve symptoms of IBS such as bloating and stomach pain.

Lung infections. Children under six who attend daycare centers seem to get fewer and less severe lung infections when given milk containing *Lactobacillus* GG or a specific combination product containing both *Lactobacillus acidophilus* and *Bifidobacterium* (HOWARU Protect).

Rheumatoid arthritis (RA). Research shows that taking *Lactobacillus casei* for eight weeks reduces tender and swollen joints in women with RA.

What to look out for when buying a probiotic:

A high colony-forming units (CFU) count

Your microbiome contains around forty trillion microbes, so to make an impact you are going to need a probiotic containing lots of bacteria. In other words, a high CFU count. Ideally you should be looking for a product that contains at least twenty billion CFUs and preferably more. Many commercial products are not even close to this minimum standard. Fermented foods are likely to hugely exceed these figures, though it is hard to generalize.

Multiple strains

Just as you want diversity in your gut, so you want a diversity of strains of microbes in your probiotic. The joy of fermented foods is that you are guaranteed diversity. If you are buying a probiotic you should be looking for one with at least six different strains.

Substrains

Lactobacillus acidophilus is not the same as *Lactobacillus casei*. If the probiotic you are thinking of buying doesn't list substrains then it may well be ineffective.

• On our website cleverguts.com we list some of the better products.

Endnotes

1   Revised estimates for the number of human and bacteria cells in the body. Sender, Fuchs, Milo, et al., *PLoS Biol*, 2016 (http://journals.plos.org/plos biology/article?id=10.1371/journal.pbio.1002533)

2   Weight loss with a low-carbohydrate, Mediterranean, or low-fat diet. Shai I et al., *New England J of Med*, 2008 (http://www.nejm.org/doi/full/10.1056 /NEJMoa0708681#t=article)

3   Successful weight loss maintenance includes long-term increased meal responses to GLP-1 and PYY 3-36. Iepsen, Lundgren, Holst, et al., *Eur J Endocrinol*, 2016 (https://www.ncbi.nlm.nih.gov/pubmed/26976129)

4   Surface area of the digestive tract revisited. Helander HF, Fandriks L, *Scandinavian J Gastroenterology*, 2014 (https://www.ncbi.nlm.nih.gov/pub med/24694282)

5   Non-celiac gluten sensitivity among patients perceiving gluten-related symptoms. Capannolo A, Viscido A, Barkad MA, et al., *Digestion*, 2015

6   A purified membrane protein from *Akkermansia muciniphila* or the pasteurized bacterium improves metabolism in obese and diabetic mice. *Nature Medicine*, 2016

7   http://www.mayoclinic.org/digestive-system/expert-answers/faq-20058340

8   Association between cesarean birth and risk of obesity in offspring in childhood, adolescence, and early adulthood. Yvan et al., *JAMA Pediatrics*, 2016

9   Environmental spread of microbes impacts the development of metabolic phenotypes in mice transplanted with microbial communities from humans. *ISME Journal*, 2016

10 Personalized nutrition by prediction of glycemic response. Zeevi et al., *Cell*, 2015

11 Is eating behavior manipulated by the gastrointestinal microbiota? Evolutionary pressures and potential mechanisms. *BioEssays*, 2014

12 Ingestion of *Lactobacillus* strain regulates emotional behavior and central GABA receptor expression in a mouse via the vagus nerve. Bravo et al., *PNAS*, 2011

13 Human metabolic phenotypes link directly to specific dietary preferences in healthy individuals. Rezzi et al., *J Proteome Res*, 2007

14   Clinical and metabolic response to probiotic administration in patients with major depressive disorder. Akkasheh et al., *Nutrition*, 2016 Mar; 32(3):315-20. doi: 10.1016/j.nut. 2015.09.003

15   The spread of obesity in a large social network over 32 years. Christakis and Fowler, *New England J of Med*, 2007 (http://www.nejm.org/doi/full/10.1056/NEJMsa066082#t=article)

16   Helminth therapy for induction of remission in inflammatory bowel disease. Garg et al., *Cochrane Database Syst. Rev*, 2014. (https://www.ncbi.nlm.nih.gov/pubmed/24442917)

17   Primary prevention of cardiovascular disease with a Mediterranean diet. Estruch et al., *New England J of Med*, 2013

18   Understanding the impact of omega-3 rich diet on the gut microbiota, Noriega et al., *Case Reports in Medicine*, 2016. (https://www.hindawi.com/journals/crim/2016/3089303/)

19   Mercury levels in commercial fish and shellfish, US Food and Drug Admin.   http://www.fda.gov/Food/FoodborneIllnessContaminants/Metals/ucm115644.htm

20   Association between omega-3 fatty acid supplementation and risk of major cardiovascular disease events: a systematic review and meta-analysis. Rizos et al., *JAMA*, 2012

21   Meta-analysis of prospective cohort studies evaluating the association of saturated fat with cardiovascular disease. Siri-Tarino et al., *Amer J of Clin Nutrition*, 2010

22   Association of dietary, circulating and supplementary fatty acids with coronary risks. Chowdhury et al., *Ann Internal Medicine*, 2014

23   Meat consumption and mortality. Rohrmann et al., *BMC Medicine*, 2013

24   Egg consumption and risk of coronary heart disease and stroke: dose-response meta-analysis of prospective cohort studies. Rong et al., *BMJ*, 2013

25   Alcohol consumption and risk of heart failure: the Atherosclerosis Risk in Communities Study. Goncalves et al., *Eur Hear J*, 2015

26   Influence of red wine polyphenols and ethanol on the gut microbiota ecology and biochemical biomarkers. Queipo-Ortuño et al., *Amer J Clin Nutr*, 2012

27   Identification of the 100 richest dietary sources of polyphenols: an application of the Phenol-Explorer database. Perez-Jimenez et al., *Eur J of Clin Nut*, 2010 (http://www.nature.com/ejcn/journal/v64/n3s/full/ejcn2010221a.html)

28   Role of curcumin in systemic and oral health: An overview. Nagpal et al., *Journal of Nat Science, Biol and Med*, 2013

29   Odorous urine following asparagus ingestion in man. Mitchell et al., *Experientia*, 1987 (https://www.ncbi.nlm.nih.gov/pubmed /3569485)

30   You're in for a treat: asparagus. Sugarman et al., *N C Med J*, 1985

31 Metabolomics investigation to shed light on cheese as a possible piece in the French paradox puzzle. Zheng et al., *Journal of Agricultural and Food Chemistry*, 2015

32 Relation between consumption of sugar-sweetened drinks and childhood obesity: a prospective, observational analysis. Ludwig et al., *Lancet*, 2001

33 Sucralose promotes food intake through NPY and a neuronal fasting response. Wang et al., *Cell Metabolism*, 2016

34 Artificial sweeteners produce the counterintuitive effect of inducing metabolic derangements. Swithers, *Trends Endocrinol Metab*, 2013

35 Artificial sweeteners induce glucose intolerance by altering the gut microbiota. Suez et al., *Nature*, 2014

36 "The conversation: your gut bacteria don't like junk food—even if you do" (https://theconversation.com/your-gut-bacteria-dont-like-junk-food-even-if-you-do-41564)

37 Dietary emulsifiers impact the mouse gut microbiota promoting colitis and metabolic syndrome. Chassaing et al., *Nature*, 2015

38 Increased gut microbiota diversity and abundance of fecal bacterium prausnitzii and Akkermansia after fasting: a pilot study. Remely et al., *Wien Klin Wochenschr*, 2015

39 What does a three-day dietary cleanse do to your gut microbiome? (http://americangut.org/what-does-a-three-day-dietary-cleanse-do-to-your-gut-microbiome/)

40 Extremely short-duration high-intensity training substantially improves the physical function and self-reported health status of elderly adults. Adamson et al., *J Am Geriatr Soc*, 2014 (https://www.researchgate.net/publication/263859177)

41 Short sleep duration, glucose dysregulation and hormonal regulation of appetite in men and women. St-Onge et al., *Sleep*, 2012

42 Fiber and saturated fat are associated with sleep arousals and slow wave sleep. St-Onge et al., *J Clin Sleep Med*, 2016

43 Neural correlates of mindfulness meditation-related anxiety relief. Zeidan F et al., *Soc Cogn Effect Neurosc*, 2014

44 Daily consumption of the collagen supplement Pure Gold Collagen® reduces visible signs of aging. Borumand and Siolla, *Clin Interv Ageing*, 2014

Acknowledgments

I would like to say a big thank you to my publishers Aurea Carpenter and Rebecca Nicolson, and the rest of the team at Short Books for their support and wise editorial advice. Also thanks to Caroline Barton for her excellent culinary contributions and to my agents Sophie Laurimore and Andrew Nurnberg for helping me get through some challenging situations. Above all, I would like to thank Clare, who has done so much to make this book possible.

Michael Mosley trained to be a doctor at the Royal Free Hospital in London. After qualifying, he joined the BBC, where he has become a well-known television host. He is the author of the internationally bestselling *FastDiet* and *The 8-Week Blood Sugar Diet*. He is married with four children.

Dr. Clare Bailey, wife of Michael Mosley, is a GP who has pioneered a dietary approach to health and reducing blood sugars and diabetes in her practice in Buckinghamshire. She is the author of *The 8-Week Blood Sugar Diet Recipe Book*, published in 2016.

Tanya Borowski is a nutritional therapist who focuses on functional medicine. She has a degree in nutritional therapy, full certification through the Institute of Functional Medicine, and specializes in treating digestive complaints such as IBS, gluten sensitivity, and celiac disease.

Index

Index

Index